A DIET FOR THE
BEER DRINKING MAN

By
Roger C. Cotta

With Commentary by
Lisa Cosman, Nutritionist

ISBN 0-7414-2780-X

Published by:

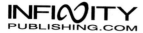
PUBLISHING.COM

1094 New DeHaven Street, Suite 100
West Conshohocken, PA 19428-2713
Info@buybooksontheweb.com
www.buybooksontheweb.com
Toll-free (877) BUY BOOK
Local Phone (610) 941-9999
Fax (610) 941-9959

Printed in the United States of America

Printed on Recycled Paper

Published May 2006

Foreword

Commentary by Lisa Cosman, Practical Nutritionist

This is a Diet Book for guys – single and married, and the wives of overweight men – written by a New Yorker, Roger Cotta, who spent much of his life eating like a baseball fan (in his younger days he was captain of his baseball team), a onetime lapsed exerciser (before this successful diet), a former U.S. Marine; generally just a regular American guy.

Roger, however, has an immense curiosity as well as a sense of pragmatism, and when extreme dieting (Atkins style) backfired on him (at it has for lots of other men), Roger researched nutrition and designed his own diet. As he tells us, he realized that he wouldn't be happy without beer – so he designed beer right into his diet (like millions of American guys, Roger seriously enjoys beer). Choosing efficiency as well as pleasure, Roger added to his weight loss dietary explorations regular exercise that he enjoys doing. Finally weight-loss dieting worked for him. At last, he took off the excess weight, then kept it off, and his cholesterol and blood pressure came down (I've verified his before and after medical records). His doctors could tell you that he has also lowered his risk for heart disease, stroke, and diabetes. Recent nutritional knowledge tells us that regular exercise and sustained good nutrition lowers the risk of Alzheimer's disease and cancer, as well.

This diet is right for beer drinking guys because it pays attention to a guy's lifestyle and taste buds. It's a diet that a man can live with and on. Roger makes no claim, nor do I (no one can in any book diet), but if you follow A Diet For The Beer-Drinking Man because it fits your body and your lifestyle, this way of dieting can make a difference for you, too.

As a New York nutritionist with decades of experience working with individuals who want to improve their health and achieve the bodies they desire, I've long realized that the diet that works for a man (or a woman) is the one they can really live with every day, a diet which contains something that feels just wicked enough that the individual can say no to excess calories and inappropriate temptations long enough to get results and to establish lasting sensible personalized eating habits; and then to maintain those new habits. The whole idea of a Beer Drinker's Diet horrifies extremists, but living realistically is not living with the denial pressure of extremism. *Roger's diet eliminates meal skipping and teaches portion control and managing carbohydrates. You can take this diet home, you can eat out.*

Since taking off weight, not only has Roger maintained his weight loss and improved medical profile, when he introduced himself to me (and first brought me the manuscript for this book) he told me that he knows now that he *will never be dangerously overweight again.* He no longer fears that.

I've gotten to know Roger, he's happy, he feels no deprivation, and his medical records speak for themselves. For you, Roger has written this book.

My question (and likely yours), *"Is this a safe diet?"*

Basically, yes (although it is definitely not the right diet for an alcoholic). Occasionally Roger still drinks rather more beer than is truly sensible (for a man, two beers a day is the medical maximum, for a woman one), but no guy starts out a paragon, they need to be trained into better habits. Roger trained himself enough to get a workable, livable diet for himself and he is a beer drinker.

I am, as well as an experienced Nutritionist and a Practical Nutritionist, a committed Wholefoodist Nutritionist. "What does that mean," you ask? I am firm about avoiding artificial foods, chemicalized foods, over processed and refined foods, and always have been; lots of vegetables (for dieters, salads with lettuces and low or medium carbohydrate raw vegetables and low-salt/no msg soups and cooked vegetables, that sort of thing; oils instead of trans fats, healthy lean protein, wholegrains, etc.)

This diet works because it is a Controlled Carbohydrate diet plan. Low-low carb diets manipulate the biochemistry and have a ruthless boomerang weight gain kick with even a small indulgence. *A Diet For The Beer-Drinking Man depends on Controlled Carbohydrates (factoring in the beer), plus portion control, consistency, regular meals, adequate sleep, and exercise.* Roger had enough sense (and his mother's voice in his ear) to take some vitamin supplements while he dieted and to get enough fiber and water *throughout the day.* We need fluids, we need fiber. *We also do need carbohydrates. Carbohydrates fuel our muscles, our hearts, and our brains.* One 1960's low-carbohydrate diet observer (he was a therapist) also noticed that excessive low-low carbohydrate eating changed people's moods negatively. We need enough carbohydrate to form serotonin, which mellows our moods (it's not just the alcohol in our beer or wine that calms us, it's their biochemical effect on our neurotransmitters). That researcher was Dr. George Watson, and his book entitled "Nutrition and The Mind", is now out of print.

Roger now rides his bicycle at least four days a week for ninety minutes on each of those days. He also plays tennis, walks frequently and stays active. He works full time, has raised a family, and is happy. He is also healthier and slimmer than during his pre Beer Drinker's Diet days. Remember, he was a U.S. Marine, a regular guy and he writes like one. You'll enjoy reading this book, and the diet is just the ticket for someone who wants to take off excess weight, but *knows* that he is not going to give up drinking beer.

This book is a good read (Roger has a very personal sense of humor) and offers a very creative diet. The author's experience will help you to discover some foods you never even dreamed you'd like; and you've still got that satisfying bit of beer. Remember, all nutritionists will tell you not to drink to excess, nor to drink if your doctor tells you not to, nor if you are pregnant or immune compromised, not even beer; nor to take up drinking if you aren't a beer drinker, now. This is a

Beer Drinker's Diet for men who drink beer. A diet that Beer Drinkers will like and that Beer Drinkers will follow.

If you picked up this book because the title grabbed you, then it's very likely the right diet book for you. I've never seen a more honest "guy's" diet book, nor any diet book less self-righteous or obsessive. This is a man's diet for real men and for the women who worry about them.

Lisa Cosman,

Nutritionist

New York City, 2006

One

Okay, so I'm a hard-core beer drinker; guzzler, swiller, gulper, call it what you like, I love my beer. For as long as I can remember, I've had three or four bottles a day. I've never tried seriously to quit, although I often wonder what my life might have been like had I not been a beer-drinker.

When asked why God created alcohol? The answer was … So that the Irish wouldn't conquer the world. Being half-Irish, perhaps I may have accomplished some phenomenal feat; even been a multi-millionaire if I never partook of spirits. I guess I won't ever know.

I can recall saying, back in the mid-seventies, when I was recently separated from my wife of thirteen years and living on Thirty-Third Street and Third Avenue in Manhattan;

"If they ever make a decent non-alcoholic beer, I'll quit drinking regular beer; because I just love the taste of it. The cold, crisp, biting taste. I don't *need* the alcohol, just the taste."

Sure.

When non-alcoholic beers hit the market, I quickly faced the realization that it was the buzz that I loved. True I loved the cold, crisp, biting taste, but I just *loved* that real beer buzz.

This is a book about how I lost some serious weight and once I lost it, kept it off and stayed at the weight I had reached. It's called the "A Diet For The Beer-Drinking Man" because every diet I've ever read about or attempted to follow, highly discourages drinking beer, wine or any kind of alcohol. From experience I've found that I've avoided trying many diets because I was unwilling to quit drinking. And when I *have* attempted to diet and coupled that with having my fill of beer or wine, I've always ended up stuffing fattening food into every appropriate orifice in my body.

Confronted by a Doctor after an intense physical, a patient who enjoyed drinking heavily was told that he would have to either quit drinking or would certainly die within the near future. The patient responded, "Can I have a few weeks to think that over?"

Like me, you who love your beer or wine know *exactly* how he felt.

I always remember a number of years back when I happened to meet a friend in the street who had just finished jogging for an hour. He was covered with sweat and his clothing was drenched. Still breathing heavily from the exercise, he pulled out a cigarette and lit up. I raised an eyebrow.

"I rationalize my smoking this way, Roger" he said. "If I *didn't* jog and smoked cigarettes, I believe that it'd be far worse for my health than jogging *and* smoking."

Similarly I believe that if I *didn't* follow this diet and still drank beer, the effects would be far more deleterious to my health.

Perhaps you may consider this a stupid statement, it certainly it wouldn't be the first one that I've uttered. Please don't think that A Diet For The Beer-Drinking Man won't work if you're not a drinker. If you don't drink now, you don't need to avoid this diet. Quite possibly, if you follow this diet and do not drink beer or wine, the resultant weight loss could be more dramatic.

The results of various studies have been reported to the effect that one who drinks in moderation, no more than three normal-sized drinks a day, will usually live longer than one who never touches a drop.

I truly loved reading that. My problem, however, was that quite frequently I would use up a full three day's rations in a single night.

The overriding premise you will read about within the following pages is that one can be *flexible* when on "A Diet For The Beer-Drinking Man". I didn't need to carefully count calories, or carbohydrates, weigh food or do whatever people do when they become almost obsessive about following a particular diet. I could substitute, cheat on occasion, even fall off for a few days and eat a few high carb meals, as long as *most of the time* I avoided high or medium-high carbohydrate foods.

As I've already stated, I drink three or four full-bodied imported beers a day, and I often substitute a few glasses of wine for a few of the beers. Regular beer is very high in carbs but regardless, I still lost the weight and kept it off.

It was about sixteen years ago when I first began reading about low-carbohydrate dieting. It all seemed quite logical and made real sense to me. Satiate yourself on any approved food; meat, fowl, fish, cheese, eggs, veggies and salad; all you want, not to worry too much about fats or cholesterol, just eat only low-carb foods and stay away from sugar, or foods that produce sugar in your body (high-carbs), such as bread, pasta, rice, potatoes, dry cereals, oatmeal, pretzels, potato chips, popcorn, cake, cookies and many high carb fruits. Also avoid certain vegetables that are high in carbs, such as most beans, tomatoes and corn.

And, of course, *stay away from alcoholic beverages.*

It was 1989 and I was then fifty-one years old. Since the early-eighties at a height of 5' 10", my weight had ranged from a low of 204 to a high of 225. I've never considered myself to be fat, just sort of overweight. I've always liked playing tennis, riding a bike and doing a lot of walking, so the extra weight never seemed to be a problem. Deep in my heart, though, I often found myself wishing that I could be slim and wonderful again just like I was in my twenties.

Like most new projects I have ever embarked upon, I started the low-carb diet *in earnest* during the fall of that year. My weight at that time was at its high of 225 and I knew that my cholesterol count was high as well. I methodically read every food label, memorized all the low-carb and high carb foods and studiously avoided eating or drinking anything that was even moderately high in carbs, except for beer.

I continued drinking coffee, although most diet-guides strongly urge you to avoid caffeine. 'Just forget about that!' I told

3

myself. It's hard enough to stick to a diet without having to suffer through caffeine withdrawal at the same time. I *love* the caffeine high, as I love the beer buzz.

As I stated earlier, I continued to drink three or four beers a night. Heretofore every low carb diet I read about highly discouraged the regular drinking of beer or alcohol. I'm a great believer in being flexible and I decided that was I simply not about to adhere to this highly restrictive diet, which cut out many of the foods that I truly loved like pasta, bread and sweets; and at the same time, deprive myself of drinking beer.

No way, Jose.

But I *did* substitute light imported beer for regular beer. As the advertisers have recently made sure to let you know, light beer is fairly low in carbs.

And guess what?

You still get the almighty buzz.

It was truly amazing!

The pounds started melting away; the theory being that if your body doesn't get the sugar it needs from your food intake, it begins to take it from your fat cells and soon begins to burn away that pesky fat which is stored in your body and you simply lose weight in the process.

It was great and I was noticeably losing weight, rarely hungry and generally feeling pretty good.

I dropped ten pounds during the first week.

I was delighted. Thrilled. Happy as a pig in a pile of mud.

Some of what I read concerning low-carb diets warned that there could be two significant side effects. First, when the lack of carbohydrates causes the body to begin burning fat which is stored inside, this process (called "ketosis") can often cause your breath to be less than acceptable. No big deal, I was then happily married to my second wife and simply decided to load up on sugar-free breath mints.

The second side effect was much harder to take.

Constipation.

For one who had never suffered with that particular problem, it was something I did *not* like. The books advised that to counter this unpleasant side effect, drink plenty of water and eat a lot of high-fiber veggies, such as broccoli and spinach. For many years I have routinely started each day with two 16 oz glasses of water, so I just began to supplement that with a few additional glasses each day. As far as eating high fiber veggies, I really love fresh spinach and I'm ambivalent about broccoli, so I followed the advice.

It didn't help much. Determined not to let this diet fail because of an annoying side effect, I bought a bottle of natural concentrated fiber pills, which is essentially fiber in tablet form. Called "Fibercon", it consists primarily of calcium polycarbophil.

I began taking two tablets a day with my morning intake of water and happily it solved the problem.

I then forged ahead with the diet and when I had lost fifteen pounds in two weeks, I felt well on my way to becoming the slim and wonderful person of my youth.

There was, however, one *deadly* side effect to the low-carb diet that the books never warned me about.

After about ten days I began dreaming in broad daylight, of some of the high carbohydrate foods that I had stricken from my diet; French fries, pasta, ziti, spaghetti, *any* kind of noodles. I was also fantasizing about bagels, english muffins, high-carb bread, bialys, kaiser rolls, croissants, Italian bread, pretzels, potato chips, you name it and I *lusted* after it.

I desperately wanted a piece of creamy cheesecake, a few scoops of ice cream, some cookies and a chocolate bar. The few meager graham crackers that I had allowed myself each day on the diet were rapidly becoming tiresome. I felt truly deprived of the foods I loved most.

What the hell, I decided, I can cheat just *one* night.

So I took a Wednesday night off from my low-carb regimen, voraciously consumed a ton of baked ziti, a loaf of Italian bread and two pieces of creamy luscious cheesecake. Before dinner I polished off six bottles of regular imported beer.

Ahhhhhhh!

So -CENSORED- good!

I was completely satisfied; like a baby after its bottle, nestled in the comfort of mommy's arms.

After all, I told myself confidently, I can easily restart the low-carb diet tomorrow.

Most assuredly.

I started the next day in earnest, taking two fiber pills and eating my low-carb foods all day. I continued for two more days and on the fourth day, once again began *fantasizing* about pasta, French fries and bread.

Fug-get-about-it.

I went home, drank six imported regular beers; ate a few juicy cheeseburgers on sesame buns, with crisp French fries; and consumed six peanut butter cups for dessert. Peanut butter cups and I go all the way back to my teenage days.

The following day I tried once again to follow the low-carb diet. Two days later I fell off the wagon again.

I tried earnestly to resume the regimen the next day.

No luck.

From then on over the next few years, I attempted to go on the low-carb diet about a half-dozen times, but to no avail. Finally I abandoned it forever, firmly convinced I could *never* stick to any low-carb diet.

At least I *thought* it was to be forever until around February of 2004 after something different and wonderful had happened to the low-carb world.

At first I paid little attention, but again and again I was reading about people who were cutting their carb intake all over the country, losing tremendous amounts of weight and keeping it off. A high profile article on low-carb eating was published in Time magazine. Included were a number of attestations from people who had enjoyed great success by cutting carbs.

'Still not for me,' I told myself dogmatically. 'I'll never be able to conquer my cravings for pasta and other carbs. No way. I just don't have that kind of strength.'

We'll soon move on to exactly how I finally managed to shed that unwanted weight while rarely feeling too hungry. You'll also read about how I got to eat a host of wonderful substitutes for high-carb foods and, best of all, was still able to drink my full-bodied beer each day; even enjoying satisfying low-carb desserts and snacks.

Hopefully you can experience this kind of success as well, with A Diet For The Beer-Drinking Man. I believe that you'll find, as I did, that there's absolutely nothing difficult about sticking to it.

Trust me, I haven't lied to you yet.

Two

I like to go out early Saturday and Sunday mornings, as well as one or two weekdays and ride my bicycle. It's the only form of formal exercise that I get. As I ride I often see these poor overweight people, jogging, fast walking, riding bikes and I just know that in many cases a lot of them are going to be stuffing their faces with a surfeit of high carb foods by lunch or dinner time.

I find myself thinking when I see these women and men with huge guts and butts, pushing themselves relentlessly in fruitless efforts to work off calories and excess fat;

'If only these unfortunate, unknowing people knew even half of what I know about successful low-carb dieting, many of them might never have to struggle with their weight again.'

One morning before I embarked upon the writing of this book, I was joking with a co-worker. I had suggested previously that he try my version of the low-carb diet and after about a week, he seemed to be doing fairly well.

"The greatest thing about this diet," I said, "is that you can still guzzle your beer."

We laughed.

"I should write a book and call it 'A Diet For The Beer-Drinking Man." I said.

"You'll sell a million copies!" he said and we roared with laughter.

As I walked away I wasn't laughing any longer. It was at that moment that I decided to write the book.

Before we actually dive into our book, let me state clearly that I am not an M.D. or PHD, or anything even remotely resembling one. I possess no advanced degrees nor do I hold any medical or nutritional specialist titles.

After participating in the raising of three children and, in the process, having to deal with almost every ailment in the book, including my own illnesses and those of my wife; I feel that I *do* know a lot about personal health from a layman's point of view. I've suffered through a number of ailments; some mildly serious; many of which were borderline psychosomatic in nature. As a result, if you tell me what's physically bothering you, the chances are that I can usually suggest a remedy that should provide you some relief.

When I was in my thirties I once experienced a sweet taste in my mouth for a few days. I called my doctor and he asked me whether I felt *any* other symptoms. I replied that I did not. He then told me not to worry.

Two minutes later I called him back and asked, "Doctor, *what kind* of other symptoms might be cause for alarm?"

He replied good-naturedly, "Roger, you don't actually think that I'm going to tell you, do you? *Guaranteed,* you'll develop one of those symptoms."

My dermatologist once commented, when confronted with one of my unusual skin ailments, "I must admit, you're extremely creative."

Honestly, I don't think that I'm a certifiable hypochondriac, but I *have* suffered a myriad of not-too serious illnesses and as a result, possess a wealth of remedies, such as mega-vitamin therapy, anti-biotics, and etcetera. Nonetheless that doesn't even come close to qualifying me as an M.D. or a medical person.

The vast majority of everything I convey to you in this book is gleaned from my personal experience. Occasionally I'll relate certain things to you that I've read, but I'll always qualify them by telling you that.

A Diet For The Beer-Drinking Man may or may not be right for you. Whatever I write here is only what I have done. I've found following this diet both easy and rewarding. I can't guaranty that you'll find success with it, but I sincerely hope you will.

That being said, let's get started.

I began with my own version of a low-carb diet in March 2004. It was almost by accident. At the time I weighed 225 pounds and my blood pressure was elevated, as was my cholesterol level. I was attempting to diet off and on, trying to stick to low-calorie and low fat foods, but with absolutely no success. I was firmly convinced that a low-carb diet would never work for me since I was a beer drinker and had tried and abandoned the diet a half-dozen times before.

I was seated in my Dentist's waiting room, leafing through a magazine and I saw an advertisement picturing a juicy hamburger with a slice of tomato, raw onion and melted cheese, wrapped in a thin, low-carbohydrate wrap, instead of a hamburger bun. I love cheeseburgers, even with low fat or fat free cheese. The idea of using a low-carb wrap instead of a bun appealed to me.

I resolved to try it that night.

With the cheeseburger and a salad, I had a delicious dinner and quickly calculated the entire carb count for the burger and salad at less than 15 grams.

A few days later, I was having lunch with a friend at a Chinese Restaurant. I wanted to try to keep the carbs down so I ordered a platter of mixed grilled crispy veggies (eggplant, cabbage, carrots, mushrooms, onions and squash, garnished with a tangy brown sauce). I passed on the white rice.

The dish was great.

I was now on my way.

From that point on I literally abandoned potatoes and rice from my diet.

To stay with the program, I began eating light bread, which is relatively low in carbs, instead of regular bread. On occasion I substituted a few slices of Melba toast or saltine crackers for the bread.

I was still alternately eating regular pasta every few nights, but of utmost importance, I had taken the first paramount step of substituting various veggies such as eggplant, mushrooms, squash and cabbage for the potatoes or rice; as well as eating light/low-carb bread instead of regular bread.

Of course I was still drinking those precious three or four regular imported beers a night.

When I embarked upon this *mix* of substituting a few low-carb foods for certain, but not all, starches, I was exercising three days a week at a health club. My exercise routine was hardly grueling, to say the least, but still it was better than nothing.

I would go to the gym each Monday, Wednesday and Friday around midday, change into my shorts and sneakers and work the stationary bicycle for twenty minutes. It usually pumped my heart rate up to between 110 and 115, which seemed more than fine for me. I broke a mild sweat and was quite happy each time I finished.

I had been doing the exercise club, coupled with real bicycle riding on the weekends, for about eighteen months. It had done little to nothing for my weight, but it had helped lower my blood pressure slightly and also made me feel better about myself.

After exercising at the club I would always step on the scale before taking a shower. When I started the diet substitution mix, I weighed 225.

After about a week I noticed that I had lost five pounds.

What? Something *must* be wrong with this scale; I told myself.

I stepped on the scale at home that night.

220. This was sensational!

From then on I progressed into eating more substitutes for carbohydrates and the weight continued to come off. I became highly motivated and even eliminated the occasional real pasta, as the weight continued to plummet. 215, 210, 205. I was feeling very good and still drinking three or four full-bodied beers every night.

When I reached 195, all of my trousers were two inches too big about the waist, my belts were too large and everyone was telling me that I had lost *a lot* of weight.

During the dramatic slide from 225 to 195, I was being super careful about avoiding carbs. On weekends I was eating breakfasts of egg whites, tuna and cottage cheese. Lunch consisted of a single glass of vegetable juice cocktail, which I mixed with lemon juice and artificial sweeteners. I substituted a sugar-free fruit drink for orange juice. Dinner was an adequate helping of meat, chicken or fish, embellished with a varied assortment of veggies and salad.

The only sweets that I allowed myself each day were a few graham crackers after dinner. The only high carb drink I partook of was my regular intake of beers.

But nonetheless, the longer that I stayed away from pasta and sweet desserts, the more I was craving them.

That was when I suddenly and happily discovered the low-carbohydrate section in my local supermarket. We'll move into that adventure in the next chapter.

A short while after reaching 195 pounds, I abandoned the stationary bicycle and the exercise club and, since the spring weather was favorable, I increased my real bike riding from just weekends, to weekends plus one or two additional mornings a week, the frequency depending upon which of me won the battle between sleeping an additional hour or dragging my lazy butt outside and mounting the bike at 5:30 a.m.

I told people that the real reason I had quit the formal exercise club program was that I had been highly embarrassed and insulted when the club's manager approached me and insisted that I wear a protective helmet while riding the stationary bicycle, because I kept falling off.

Three

Okay, let's continue with my success story. Briefly reviewing the first two chapters, I took you through my history since 1989, of unsuccessfully attempting stay on low-carb diets, for fairly simple reasons; I was not about to quit my daily regimen of beer drinking. I felt that I was also too weak to resist the starch and high carb food cravings that, for me, always accompanied low-carb dieting.

In March of 2004, just around the time of my son's eighteenth birthday, I tried the cheeseburger in a low-carb wrap and discovered veggie substitutes for potatoes and pasta.

By July, after sticking to low-carb substitutes for bread and potatoes, my weight had plummeted from 225 to 195. I felt that the thirty-pound loss was enough for the time being, so I decided to try to simply maintain that weight. I was still, however, fantasizing about eating ziti or spaghetti; bagels with cream cheese; potato chips; cookies; cheesecake and candy.

So I began to cheat slightly, eating some of these high carb foods two or three nights a week while sticking to the low-carb regimen the other nights. Unhappily I noticed that some of the weight began to come creeping back.

I *simply had* to find an acceptable substitute for noodles, which was the food that I most strongly craved; after all, my roots are half-Italian. I tried shredded tofu, which looks a bit like spaghetti noodles, but does not come near doing the trick. No matter how long or short one cooks it, the texture was never soft enough. I recalled seeing soy noodles in my supermarket. I bought some and quickly abandoned them, since again they could not be cooked soft enough for this desperate camper's particular taste. They were also a dark brownish color, which didn't quite sit right with me.

One day I stumbled upon the new low-carbohydrate section in my supermarket. There were thin spaghetti and penne noodles; low-carb bread of varied flavors; an array of all kinds of low-carb cookies and low-carb ice cream, puddings, candy bars and yogurt. There were even Soya cheddar cheese chips and barbeque flavored Soya chips. While low-carb wraps had been available for a few months, they stocked them as well; and I found a relatively low-carb pecan granola cereal, which was quite delicious, high in fiber and really helped as a dessert substitute.

And guess what? In the frozen section there was even a low-carb low fat *cheesecake*.

I gaped at the revelation, a virtual "Stranger in Paradise".

I stocked up on samples of everything.

Happily, I tried the low-carb penne noodles that very same night and to my delight, they cooked to a delectable softness.

I served the noodles topped with red lobster sauce and a few shrimps, buttered two slices of low-carb bread and absolutely felt like crying, I was so thrilled.

Never again would I crave noodles or bread.

The Soya cheddar cheese chips actually tasted better to me than real potato chips, with the added benefit of having no trans-fatty acids and were low in fat as well as carbs.

The cookies weren't bad either and while the cheesecake wasn't your typical New York creamy cheesecake, it still helped to satisfy the urge.

From then on I was in business.

My creativity took over and I learned how to substitute low-carb foods for almost everything except bagels, which I still craved for.

Fortunately a month later, low carb bagels popped up in bagel stores and some supermarkets began to carry some more varieties of low-carb wraps. God had smiled upon me.

I dropped another 5 pounds without even thinking. I could now easily maintain my new slim (and wonderful?) self at 190 pounds.

You may recall the canned nutritional vanilla and chocolate shakes, fortified with vitamins and minerals, that popped up a number of years ago, as a popular and effective substitute for one or two meals a day. The advertising campaigns were huge. Celebrities were attesting as to how much weight they had lost. People all over the country were substituting these low fat, relatively low calorie shakes for their high calorie morning bagels and cream cheese, or buttered rolls; as well as their high fat high calorie luncheon sandwiches, hamburgers or whatever else they stuffed themselves with. By doing this, while eating a normal dinner and moderately drinking wine or beer, people began losing weight on the nutritional shake program.

You ask, how?

They were substituting the lower calorie shakes for their high calorie breakfasts and lunches. The only problem with this program was that, like anything taken repeatedly, the nutritional shakes lacked real variety. It was easy to become bored with them. Of course the manufacturers aggressively attempted to combat this with the introduction of other nutritional meal substitutes such as soups, snacks and cookies, but these simply never enjoyed the initial successes that the shakes had.

Two women at lunch were discussing nutritional shakes and one commented, "I just love those vanilla shakes. They're especially delicious with a large scoop of strawberry ice cream!"

Replacement of high carb foods with low-carb foods works best when there is creative variety in the substitutions. In following chapters we'll discuss that *necessary* variety and how it can help satisfy a host of cravings, such as those for Italian foods, Japanese dishes, Chinese take out foods, potatoes, rice, sandwiches and even Pizza pie.

In other sections, we'll cover exercise and its value both physically and more important, emotionally. We'll also discuss vitamins and other supplements and how they can help you live longer and healthier. I'll present my views on fats, cholesterol and trans-fatty acids; as well as drinking in moderation and how you can modify your habits and still remain satisfied.

As you can surmise by holding this relatively thin book, there is not a plethora of written word between its covers. Aside from the anecdotes that I insert at appropriate and sometimes, even inappropriate spots to keep you grinning, most of my book covers a few simple subjects; How I got going on A Diet For The Beer-Drinking Man, managed to stick with it and maintained the weight that I'm comfortable with.

You will note that I used the term "how I", instead of "how you". The reason is simple as I stated earlier. While personally I've been successful with this diet, I'm not saying or even suggesting that it will work for you.

But then again, why *shouldn't* it work for you? It worked for me and I'm just a normal person (although I could easily name a dozen individuals who will strongly disagree with that statement). And you, with your special talents and abilities, your wonderful hopes and dreams, your inner and outer beauty and kindness, are nonetheless another normal person as well.

Four

From this point on it was fairly easy. Each day, upon arising I routinely start with two 16 oz glasses of water. This has been my habit since I was a lowly recruit in the United States Marine Corps in 1956, going through training at Parris Island, South Carolina. We attended lectures on a variety of subjects, one of which was proper physical hygiene. A good percentage of the recruits were from the deepest parts of the south and, while not to be generally disparaging of southerners, some of these good ole boys had hardly worn shoes before and were accustomed to bathing in a nearby river or stream once or twice a month.

We were instructed as to how to properly clean ourselves, not missing any parts of the body while showering; how to powder our feet to avoid athlete's foot, brush the teeth, even the proper way to clean our ears.

The Staff Sergeant conducting the classes would always begin with, "A good Marine is lean and mean and a good Marine is clean!"

He told us we should begin each day with two or three large glasses of water.

"You eat a big dinner and then you don't usually have too much activity until you hit the sack. You lie in bed all night and much of that food slowly works its way down from your stomach to your digestive system, then it just sits around in your intestines for the rest of the night. There's all this nasty waste and poisons that the body has chosen not to absorb, simply hangin' around inside you.

When you drink those two or three glasses of water in the morning, you flush away all that junk and start the day with clean insides."

It certainly made a lot of sense to me.

This has absolutely nothing to do with dieting but its one of my all-time favorite true stories. It was brought to mind when I started thinking about the hygienic lectures in the Marines.

I can remember with vivid clarity, the day that I stayed a bit too long in the shower.

At boot camp the shower room was similar to those that you see in a gym or in a high school; a large tiled room with shower spigots every three feet, providing about thirty spots for the recruits to shower.

There were over eighty recruits in our platoon and we were usually allowed only eight to ten minutes for all of us to shower and be back in front of our bunks, dressed in our underwear, ready for sleep.

Showering was pure pandemonium. Imagine over eighty naked bodies clamoring for space under only thirty showerheads and every one of us trying to be back at our bunks, dried and changed into our underwear within eight to ten minutes.

This particular evening somehow I lost control of the time and as I was happily washing myself under the hot spray of water, I suddenly began to realize that I was completely alone in the shower room.

I turned off the water, took my soap, and nervously looked outside for my towel, which I had left on a hook. Someone had grabbed it.

Jesus! I thought. If the Drill Instructor catches me running naked to my bunk, without a towel wrapped around my midsection, I'm dead meat!

My heart stopped as I approached the double doors leading to the barracks. The Drill Instructor was in the center of the squad bay seated on a table and the entire platoon was gathered around him. Some of the recruits were in their underwear and others still had towels wrapped about their mid-section.

The D.I. was talking to the platoon about recent developments in the mid-east, namely the then turbulent situation in Burma, where the Chinese had just occupied 1,000 square miles after a few border clashes. Everyone was listening raptly to the

Sergeant who was seated with his back to the door; a full twenty feet inside the squad bay.

I opened one of the doors quietly, crept inside and began to make my way stealthily along the open space between the row of bunks and the wall. When I was halfway through the barracks and almost at my bunk, the D.I.'s voice boomed;

"Private Cotta!"

I froze.

"Get your naked butt, front and center, Boy!"

I complied and within a few seconds I was standing stark naked in front of the D.I. and the rest of the platoon.

"Private Cotta," he said savoring the moment. "Just exactly where is your towel?"

"Sir!" I bellowed standing at attention. "Someone must've taken it, Sir!"

A murmur of laughter trickled from the other recruits.

"Now Private Cotta," the D.I. continued, "just what makes you think you could sneak in here without me seein' you? You thought you was hidin' behind that big appendage of yours, but I seen you anyway!"

Okay, let's get back to the diet, shall we? First we'll talk about your breakfast.

This next paragraph is very important.

As you read through the following selections bear in mind that each item (e.g. an omelet or a sandwich) counts as one or two choices. For breakfast or lunch you are permitted no more than a total of *two choices* for the entire meal. Also, please don't attempt to memorize or write each selection down. You'll find a convenient listing of all of your choices in the final pages of the book.

You need not write down any recipes or earmark the pages, since the major recipes are listed at the end of each of the food selection chapters, with an alphabetical index at the end of the book.

As a starter, you can have any style of eggs including fried, boiled or scrambled (preferably a fat-free egg substitute); or alternatively you may wish to have 6 hard-boiled egg-whites, which are quite delicious with a sprinkle of parmesan or Romano cheese. I also like to lightly cover hard-boiled egg whites, or scrambled eggs, with the powdered cheese that can be found in a box of macaroni and cheese. It comes in a separate package inside the box of macaroni noodles. Read the label and make sure that the cheese contains no partially hydrogenated oils; most do not. I keep it in a saltshaker and also use it on veggies and low-carb noodles as well.

Another choice can be any kind of an omelet, made with whole eggs, egg whites or a fat-free egg substitute. The omelet can be made adding any low-carb food including ham or cheese. An omelet by itself or with veggies, mushrooms or onions, counts as a single choice. With added cheese or ham it counts as two. If you fry the eggs or omelet try to use cooking oil sparingly, or else a light oil spray. Cooking oil is low in carbs but who needs that added fat? A certain amount of fat is essential for your diet but you don't need to overdo it.

As an alternate breakfast selection you can choose from many kinds of cheese, up to three slices, with not too much fat please; also cottage cheese, farmer's cheese or up to three thin slices of ham or turkey.

Do you like tuna, egg, chicken or seafood salad? You can elect to have 4 to 6 oz of your choice. Try to make it with mayo that is made with expeller pressed oils, which tastes just as good as regular mayonnaise and contains no partially hydrogenated oils or trans fatty acids. If you cannot find this mayo in the supermarket, you can or look for it in your local health food store. If you still can't find it simply use low fat mayo. You can also creatively embellish the salads with chopped celery, scallions, green peppers and onions, if you wish.

Cholesterol free egg salad can be made by cooking a small amount of egg substitute then chopping it up with hard-boiled egg whites and celery and mixing with low fat mayo.

What I've shown you thus far in this chapter, as selections for your breakfast, are more in line with the traditional breakfasts you are used to eating and those that I personally allow myself.

Other choices include low-carb yogurt, approved veggies and certain relatively low-carb fruits. Keep the portions moderate and make sure they are all low-carb foods. *Avoid most fruit juices unless they are truly low in carbs and I know of few that actually are.* Supermarkets now carry a few fruit punch drinks which are sweetened with Splenda and contain only 3 grams of carbs per 8 oz serving. There are a number of sugar free fruit drinks that contain zero carbs. Tropicana also makes a "Light" orange juice that is delicious and relatively low in carbs.

Yes, you can have toast as long as it is no more than two slices of low-carb bread; or else three slices of Melba toast, or five fat-free saltine crackers. Each counts as one choice.

Relatively low-carb bagels are now available in most bagel stores and supermarkets are carrying whole-grain mini-bagels and English muffins which are also comparatively low in carbs. They should, however, be taken only on occasion, *until your weight loss is under your control*, since a single "low carb bagel or English can contain up to 18 grams of carbs.

Butter is fine with the toast. Actually I prefer light margarine made with expeller-pressed oils; as with the mayo, it contains no trans-fatty acids or partially hydrogenated oils, is lower in saturated fat and has zero cholesterol. Cream cheese is also okay, but not a big schmeer; again try to find that made with expeller pressed oils, usually available in health food stores. Bagel and health-food stores now sell a Tofu spread, which is free of cholesterol and tastes great.

For those of you who feel the need for high fiber in the morning, you can satisfy that with the natural fiber pill

21

supplements mentioned in chapter one. There also are plenty of other commercial fiber supplements that work equally as well.

If, however, you would like to eat a high fiber bran cereal, some "extra fiber" bran cereals contain as little as 7 grams of carbs per serving. An ounce two of skim milk won't add appreciably to the carb count.

Avoid the commercial dry cereals that claim to be high in fiber, they are usually loaded with carbs; unless, of course, the carb count is 10 grams or less.

Take at least one 12 oz glass of water or other liquid (preferably 1 ½ glasses) with any high fiber cereal. It's very important to remember when taking a high fiber food or supplement, *that you need to drink plenty of liquid at the same time*. Fiber expands in the intestines and can cause a blockage without enough liquid.

Diet drinks, flavored seltzer or other low-carb drinks *do not count* as choices, but please don't drink a lot of diet soda. Currently most diet drinks are sweetened with aspartame, which is okay in moderation, but should not be consumed in excess. There is of late, a slow trend toward sweetening diet drinks with Splenda, which many feel is preferable to aspartame. Flavored or unflavored seltzer has zero carbs and can be consumed without restriction as you would plain water. Coffee and tea have no carbs and adding a small amount of milk adds minimally to that.

I like to make a vegetable juice cocktail to drink with breakfast and other meals. It is relatively low in carbs and sodium and has the added benefit of lemon juice. To prepare it simply buy a 46-ounce bottle or can of vegetable juice, which is preferably, *but not essentially*, low in sodium. Take an empty bottle of the same size (46 oz.) and empty half of the vegetable juice into it. Then pour three ounces of reconstituted lemon juice into each of the two bottles (for more or less tang, modify the amount of lemon juice). Fill the remainder with filtered water. Add a few packets of Splenda or any *non-aspartame* sweetener according to your taste (you can find some good natural non-sugar sweeteners such as Stevia in health food stores). Shake the mixture well and chill.

The raw carbs and sodium have been cut in half to 4 grams per 8 oz serving, by adding the lemon juice and water. The beverage has a very pleasant tang, without having the rich texture that you normally associate with tomato or vegetable juices.

Regardless of what you select, the main thing to remember about breakfast is to eat moderate portions. You can satisfy your hunger easily with a maximum of two choices selected from the above paragraphs and still walk away from the table with the knowledge that you've had a good low-carb breakfast.

If you want to be creative you can take one *full* choice and two *one-half* choices, still totaling *two*. As an example, select hard-boiled eggs (one choice) or else tuna salad (one choice). Add two oz of cottage cheese (one-half choice) and a single slice of low-carb toast (one-half choice). So by cutting two of the choices in *half*, you've increased your total number of selections to three but still kept it within the total limit of two.

Am I a tricky devil?

Please understand that you can create your own menus from the previous paragraphs, or you can select from the "Breakfast Choices" section in the last few pages of the book. The segment lists each selection, its recommended proportions and the number to its right (in parenthesis), either a (1) or (2), tells you how many choices this selection counts for.

I usually drink a cup of coffee upon arriving in the office and a cup in mid-afternoon. I have continued this practice on the diet. Artificial sweeteners are okay together with a small amount of milk. Many diets discourage caffeine, but this kid *needs his caffeine jumpstart* in the morning and later on in the day.

I'll close this chapter with a final thought. As with most diets, even low-carb diets, as long as you're getting all of the nutrients your body needs, you can eat less and lose weight quicker. The traditional conception of low-carb diets is that, during any meal, you can allow yourself a surfeit of any approved food.

I don't approve of gorging oneself on any kind of food.

If you wish to take generous portions of approved veggies, that's okay; *but don't get carried away with huge portions of other foods.* I offer that you should lose weight much quicker if you keep your portions at *moderate* levels. Portion control is always important, even on a low-carb diet.

A number of years back I worked with two fine young gentlemen, who were both married and beginning to experience weight problems. I suggested that they try a low-carb diet. Each day I noticed that they were avoiding breads or pasta and rice, but they were literally loading up on meats. Without exaggeration, they would each consume well over a pound of roast pork, lamb, beef, chicken and whatever else, until they felt satiated.

Needless to say, their low-carb diets didn't last too long.

I hope that you're having at least half of the fun reading this book as I had in writing it. Hang in; we have a lot more good stuff for you. Over following chapters we'll talk about lunch.

Cholesterol Free Egg Salad

Ingredients:

4 oz of "Egg Beaters" or any Fat-Free egg substitute

6 whole eggs

1 or 2 stalks of celery

2 to 4 tablespoons of Mayonnaise made with expeller pressed oils, or any cholesterol-free mayonnaise.

Directions:

Cook the Egg Beaters in a microwave or non-stick frying pan.

Chop up the cooked Egg Beaters.

Boil the 6 whole eggs until hard.

Remove the whites and discard the yolks (the puppy will love them).

Chop up the whites and the celery.

Mix the chopped Egg Beaters, the egg whites and the celery with the mayonnaise.

Add salt and pepper to taste.

Omelets

Ingredients:

Whole eggs, or egg whites or fat free egg substitute.

Veggies, mushrooms, fresh spinach (and optionally, ham or cheese)

Cooking oil spray

Directions:

Spray a large skillet with oil. Heat under high until pan is very hot.

Pour in the eggs. Cover and reduce heat to low. After about two minutes, the eggs should be fairly well cooked.

Sprinkle with the veggies, mushrooms and/or fresh spinach. If you are adding ham or cheese, lay the slices over the eggs at this point.

Using a spatula, slide it underneath one-half of the omelet and carefully flip the half over until the omelet is in a half-moon shape.

Cover and cook *on low* for another one to 1 ½ minutes.

As described above the omelet is one choice. If you add ham or cheese, the choices become two.

Roger's Vegetable Juice Cocktail

Ingredients:

46 oz. Bottle of regular or low-sodium vegetable juice cocktail or Tomato Juice

6 oz of bottled lemon or lime juice

2 to 4 packets of artificial sweetener (Splenda, Equal, Sweet and Low, or Stevia, a natural sweetener.)

Directions:

Put half of the 46 oz of juice (23 oz) in a empty 46 oz container. Add 2 oz the lemon or lime juice to each container. Fill the remainder of each container with water.

Add two (or less according to your taste) packets of the sweetener to each container and shake. Yields two 46 oz containers of the cocktail.

By dilution, the carbs are cut in half to 4 grams per 8 oz serving.

Reduce or increase the tartness by modifying the amount of lemon or lime juice.

Five

I've undertaken a number of different exercise programs in the past forty years. I can recall that the very first one was after I had been married for two years and had put on a fair amount of weight. I was working downtown at the time and went to an exercise club in the Woolworth Building on my lunch hour. The manager gave me an impressive tour of the facilities. He informed me that I would be assigned a personal trainer. They took my blood pressure, listened to my lungs and concluded that I was, while a bit overweight, in reasonably good health. I wrote them a check for a hundred dollars for the first few months, signed a membership form and agreed to come by after work for my first session. I was asked to bring sneakers, shorts, and a jockstrap, soap, a towel and shower slippers.

I showed up at six p.m. rip-roaring and ready to go. They introduced me to Dan who was to be my personal trainer. As I looked at Dan, I was reminded uncomfortably of one of my Marine Corps drill instructors. Over the ensuing half-hour the man ruthlessly put me through an incredibly rigorous series of exercises, including accelerated treadmill jogging, as well as far too many pushups and sit-ups.

For one who was fairly out of shape and had not consciously exercised for over six years since the Marine Corps, this grueling workout was just too much for me. After awhile I was forced to stop, trying to catch my breath. I felt light headed and dangerously close to fainting.

Dan gaped at me as though seeing a leper and told me to take it easy for a while. He disappeared and I never saw him again.

After I had taken a shower, the club's manager showed up smiling and handed me my check for one hundred dollars. Sorry, he said, they had made a big mistake in allowing me to sign up. Unfortunately there were no available memberships and as a matter of fact, they had been full to capacity for over a week. If I

28

wanted to call them in a few weeks they would let me know when the next opening was.

Of course I was young and naïve at the time and believed what he told me. Feeling down, I went home and related how I had been booted out of the club, to my first wife, Barbara, who was a very smart woman.

"Schmuck." she said grinning. "They were afraid you'd have a heart attack and die right there in the club!"

The lesson to be learned is that no matter what kind of an exercise program you embark upon, be careful to start off very slowly. Don't push yourself. Gradually build up your wind and your capacity.

For a variety of reasons, primarily the lack of proper motivation, I was never successful with exercise programs at gyms. I found the treadmill or stationary bike to be incredibly boring, even if I read or watched T.V. at the time.

Over the years I've purchased various items for home exercise; a rowing machine, stationary bicycle, stair-climber-master and stationary skiing machine. Each unit eventually ended up gathering dust in my basement and was eventually thrown out because it took up too much space.

The only thing that I really found useful and that I have continued to use is a regular bicycle. For years, I have ridden an hour each day on Saturday's and Sundays. During each additional day off from work I took an extra ride. For me riding a bicycle outside is the only method of exercise that I have not found boring.

During the past year, I stepped up the bicycle a bit, adding twenty minutes to the duration and one or two extra mornings a week. It's truly a wonderful feeling to get out on the roads early in the morning when other people are sleeping and ride like the wind. When you're finished you feel as though you've really accomplished something. Assuming I'm physically able, I fully expect to be regularly riding the bicycle for as long as I live.

Some people swear by their gym. To them it's an organized, structured program they can follow two to three days a week and stay in shape. Others enjoy aerobics, where they can dance and gyrate about wildly to rhythmical music and a hard driving instructor. Some love jogging, which I have tried over the years. To me it was almost as good as bicycle riding, but eventually my knees gave out and I was forced to stop.

Even a regular routine of brisk walking three or four times a week for an hour at a time, is an excellent form of exercise.

There are two things that instill similar feelings of reluctance in me when preparing to do them. The first is going to church. The second is going to the exercise club. For many people, it's a drag to get yourself to either place, but when it's over, you feel really good.

I've often thought, wouldn't it be great if they had stationary exercise bicycles in church instead of wooden benches? After entering, everyone takes his or her place on an exercise bike and begins immediately to peddle. The bikes would be electronically wired so that once one sits on the seat an embarrassing loud alarm goes off if you don't peddle continuously.

There are only two times during the service that one is permitted to cease peddling. The first time is when the pastor or priest delivers his sermon. By the time he begins to speak, you're so delighted to be able to take a rest that you're actually *happy to listen.*

The next peddling break comes about twenty minutes later, when the weekly collection is being taken.

Did you ever think that you'd be happy to hear a sermon and give away your money?

Of course when you've finished you feel great. In a single hour you've gotten both your weekly exercise and religious service out of the way. You killed the two proverbial birds.

Regardless of what kind of a regular exercise program you choose, it can have enormously good effects upon your blood pressure, your general physical state of health and on your mental attitude.

If you don't currently exercise, I strongly urge you to consider it. Get a check up from your G.P. and make sure there are no existing health problems that should prevent you from exercising.

Again even a brisk walk for twenty or thirty minutes each day is great.

Once you find the right regimen for you, you'll feel wonderful and hopefully continue for the rest of your healthy life.

Six

Please forgive the pun, but now we're beginning to get into the meat of this diet. We're ready to cover lunches.

I can recall a number of years back I knew a lovely woman who had a weight problem. We worked together and became friends. After a while we drifted apart and when we hooked up again it was for lunch. During our separation she had lost a substantial amount of weight and looked truly wonderful.

We both ordered Chef's salads. When ordering she told the waitress, "No ham, croutons or cheese and just oil and vinegar on the side, please."

By the time I had wolfed down my entire salad and was scraping the plate clean, she was less than a third finished and picking away listlessly at the remainder.

"Do you know what, Roger?" she said, "There are times that I even *forget* to eat a meal."

"Really?" I asked.

"And I don't even realize I've missed it, until its time for the next meal."

"Do you know what I have to say to all that, Sweetie?" I asked her.

"What?"

"Screw you."

This woman wasn't actively dieting at the time, so if she missed a meal it didn't throw her off of the routine of her diet. Until your weight loss is totally under your control *it's not a good idea to skip a meal* simply because you may not be feeling hungry. The result could be that you wake up in the middle of the night, famished, and over-indulge in high-carb snacks.

Remember that this diet is designed to keep your hunger satisfied. In the beginning, you'll need all three meals to do that.

You can eat a complete lunch every day of the week as long as it's a low-carb lunch. That means limiting your lunch to one sandwich or a hamburger or grilled chicken, on a low-carb wrap, light or low-carb bread.

As far as what you can put inside the sandwich, certainly two to three thin slices of any cold cut meat or low-fat cheese is fine; as well as tuna, chicken, seafood or egg salads, made with expeller pressed mayo or mustard, as described in the breakfast menu. I like broiled or grilled eggplant slices with lettuce, a thin slice of tomato and mayo; it makes a delicious sandwich. Just keep the thin tomato slice to just one and pile on the lettuce. Fried egg whites on low-carb bread or wrap with lettuce and mayo, is quite tasty as well.

Hamburgers or grilled chicken sandwiches are superb, served on a low-carb wrap, with a very thin slice of tomato, raw onion and one slice of low fat cheese. A hamburger or grilled chicken counts as two choices, with or without the cheese. A bit of ketchup or mayo is fine.

Grilled chicken on a low-carb wrap or bread is also great, with mayo, one thin slice of tomato, lettuce and one slice of cheese.

Of course, another option is to eat a traditional salad with low-carb dressing and without croutons.

You might also elect to have a bowl of thin soup *without* noodles, rice or corn. Consume or Miso soup is a single choice even with added mushrooms, veggies, tofu or eggplant. Happily, French onion soup contains reasonably few carbs, even with mozzarella cheese, but forget about the traditional chunk of floating French bread. All cream soups should be avoided, as they are fairly high in carbs, as is tomato or pea soup.

Hey! What about Pizza?

Spread out one large low-carb wrap (or a large pita, sliced flat-wise) on a pizza tin or a sheet of aluminum foil. Spoon a *thin* coating of Italian sauce over the wrap and a sprinkle of oregano. You can also use the commercial bottled pizza sauces. Cover with a layer of low fat shredded mozzarella cheese (and one tsp. of parmesan cheese, then a thin spray of olive oil. If you wish you can garnish with sliced pepperoni, mushrooms, black olive slices, onions, peppers or anything else you desire. Bake at 425 until the cheese is crispy and brown.

Be innovative for lunch.

Keep your total carbs as low as you can. You can eat up to two choices and bear in mind that one slice of light or low-carb bread counts as one-half choice.

As a drink; coffee, tea, flavored seltzer, diet iced tea or diet soda is fine. Even a bottle of *non-alcoholic* or light beer is okay.

Sorry but no desserts yet, even low-carb, they are permitted after dinner as a reward for you for having been so wonderfully Spartan as to have adhered to your diet all day.

Again, for those who like to refer to a chart, I have constructed a "Luncheon Choices" list located at the end of the book.

I recall watching the Johnny Carson show one night many years back. He called out his premier guest of the evening, the renowned comedian, Buddy Hackett. For those of you who are too young to have caught Buddy's act, he was always a truly funny man and even his natural speech patterns made you laugh. For most of his career he was fairly overweight.

When he came on, it was evident that he had lost a significant amount of poundage. He looked terrific.

Johnny said, "God, Buddy, look at you! How much weight did you lose?"

"About 50 pounds," the comedian replied proudly.

The audience broke into wild applause.

"Tell us Buddy," Johnny urged, "how did you do it?"

"Well Johnny, I went for almost three months eating nothing but a single hard-boiled egg a day."

"Wow!" the host replied with amazement. "Nothing else?"

"Only water."

More applause.

"Come on Buddy," Johnny asked, "no alcohol?"

"Not a drop!"

"You are one amazing guy! Tell me, why'd you go on such a strict diet?"

"Well, I wanted to look good for women."

Laughter.

"You look absolutely marvelous!"

"But I'll tell you Johnny," Buddy continued reflectively, "after three months of just eating a single egg a day, I totally *forgot* what women were for."

Buddy's diet, albeit quite restrictive, was truly low-carb. The egg is one of nature's perfect foods. It supplies protein, needed fat and is very low in carbs; but a diet comprised solely of eggs does not provide all of the essential nutrients necessary to keep one in good health.

There was a measure of truth in Buddy's last comment about forgetting what women were for. If you don't get the proper nutrients, improper dieting can seriously affect your health and your emotional state. As it turned out Buddy was also taking a strong therapeutic multi-vitamin, mineral supplement, which helped stave off some of the negative effects of his diet.

The book's following chapters cover dinner and desserts, interspersed with chapters on vitamins and other natural supplements; and moderate drinking.

I trust that you've already started on the diet and I hope you're finding it as easy and user friendly as I have.

Low Carb Sandwich

Ingredients:

Low carb bread, light bread, or low carb wrap

Lettuce and 1 thin slice of tomato

Mayonnaise, preferably made with expeller pressed oils. Short of this, a low fat mayo, or

Dijon mustard

3 thin slices of any cold cut, or

3 thin slices of cholesterol free cheese (veggie cheese is good), or

3 slices combined of cold cuts and cheese, or

A shrimp, chicken, tuna or seafood salad made with mayo (expeller pressed oils)

Directions:

Make as you would otherwise make any sandwich.

Hamburger or Grilled Chicken Sandwich

Ingredients:

1 low carb wrap

4 oz lean chopped beef or

4 oz of boneless chicken breast

1 slice low fat cheese

1 slice of raw onion (hamburger only)

1 very thin slice of tomato

1 tablespoon of ketchup (hamburger) or mayo (grilled chicken)

Directions:

Pan fry or grill the burger

Or grill the chicken

Serve in a wrap with the above listed embellishments.

Pizza

Ingredients:

One large sized low carb wrap

Pizza sauce (usually sold in 12 oz jars)

Shredded low fat mozzarella cheese 4 to 6 oz

One tablespoon Parmesan cheese

Olive oil spray

Directions:

Spread the large wrap on a pizza baking tin or a sheet of aluminum foil

Cover with a thin coating of sauce

Sprinkle on the Parmesan cheese

Sprinkle on the mozzarella cheese

Spray on a thin coating of olive oil

Bake at 450 until the cheese is brown and crispy

Seven

As we all know, there are numerous ways to lose weight. In the early sixties, when I had gained far too much after only two years of marriage, my doctor prescribed a Benzedrine-based diet pill, to be taken once in the morning and again in late afternoon.

Did it work!

I lost thirty-five pounds during the first month and had never felt such an incredible sense of high energy in my life. I found that for about two to three hours after taking the pill I felt as though there was nothing in the world that I couldn't accomplish. I was also talking non-stop to co-workers; and while I realized that I was doing it, I was powerless to control it.

I was working furiously, putting out double my normal daily output. At nights, I was writing a novel at the time and the pages literally poured out of me. At eleven at night, I found myself vacuuming or cleaning the apartment.

After the first thirty-day prescription ran out, I got a refill and continued on my high. I no longer cared about losing weight; just about the magnificent high I was feeling when taking the diet pills.

When the next thirty-day refill ran out I called my Doctor and asked him for another refill. He told me that he wanted to see me before prescribing any more diet pills. After examining me and congratulating me for my forty-pound weight loss, he said that I had lost enough and should now try to stabilize my weight. He gave me a diet to follow and said that he wanted to see me in a month.

Whoa! I thought. "Doctor, what about my prescription renewal?" I asked meekly.

"What for?" he asked.

"To help me stabilize," I offered meekly.

"Roger, you shouldn't need anything other than to maintain your current eating habits."

"But,...Doctor,..." I stammered, "I don't know if I *can* maintain without the help of the pills."

"Nonsense!" he said, standing and ushering me out of the office. "See you in a month."

At first, without the pills, life hardly seemed seem worth living. I missed my daily highs, my boundless energy. Nonetheless I managed to survive.

Of course the weight came back, but eventually I realized that I had been on the borderline of becoming addicted to those lovely diet pills, so I never went back to them.

I tried over-the-counter diet pills and they worked for a while, but I found that the active ingredient in them was making my heart palpitate, so I steered clear of them as well.

At one stage I even tried hypnosis. I attended a group session with about twenty others and after the instructor successfully put the majority of the group under hypnosis, we all came to, realizing to our amazement that over twenty minutes had suddenly elapsed and we had no recollection as to what had transpired during that time.

The instructor, a woman in her forties, told us that we could come for six weekly sessions, for a five-hundred and seventy-five dollar fee and that we should almost all lose weight.

After careful consideration I decided against the weekly sessions. I had observed that the instructor was somewhat overweight. Now if this woman couldn't control her own weight, how on Earth was she going to show us how to control ours?

Liquid protein diets, Slim-Fast, Metrecal, Natural Diet Pills, I think I tried almost everything at one point or another. While they may have been great for millions of people, somehow, nothing ever seemed to work for me. The only time that I was able to lose weight effectively was when I had met a new love in my life and strongly desired to get her into bed. The motivation was there all right, but somehow after I achieved that goal, the desire to lose weight dissipated.

My mother, may she rest in peace, left me with the one of the greatest legacies I have received in life. When I was sixteen she told me that I should begin taking a regular daily strong vitamin/mineral supplement. She had been reading in a number of different publications that we don't get enough essential vitamins and minerals merely from the food that we eat. She felt that I should start taking them early in life rather than later.

Since it was 1956 at the time and the general consensus was that you don't really need to take vitamins as long as you "eat right", this was fairly progressive thinking on my Mother's part.

So I took myself to the nearest Whelan drug store and asked the pharmacist for a strong multivitamin/mineral supplement. He handed me a bottle of something therapeutic and said,

"This'll bring back that old vim and vigor!"

I suppressed my laughter and paid for the pills and I've been taking strong multivitamin/minerals ever since then.

To some extent that has contributed to the fact that, in my late-sixties, I have virtually no wrinkles on my face, have all of my teeth and my health is excellent. I thank the Lord I have never had a serious illness in my life.

Of course I must attribute my good health to a number of other factors as well. First, I don't smoke and have always attempted to exercise, albeit in irregular spurts, but still more often than not. Second, I have diverse interests, which keep me active and constantly working at something or other. Third, I get plenty of sleep, try to eat right and generally take good care of myself.

But I feel that the vitamin/mineral supplements have clearly helped. Over the years I have supplemented the one-daily vitamin/mineral tablet, by adding some additional vitamins and natural supplements.

First, I'm a strong believer in the anti-oxidant theory. That is, that a combination of vitamin C, E and Beta Carotene, taken regularly can prevent cancer. Ever since vitamins C and E became the rage in the seventies, I have taken an additional 500 mg of C and 200 mg of E. My therapeutic multivitamin/mineral tablet contains Beta Carotene, so I felt I was getting a good anti-oxidant combination. Of course C and E have other beneficial effects for your immune system, etc. In case you are one of the rare individuals who are sensitive to Vitamin C, try Ester C, which doesn't seem to upset the system.

Years ago I had some recurring knee problems, which caused me to quit jogging. Once I even developed a bad knee while simply walking normally. I went to a specialist and he immediately wanted to schedule me for an operation. Since the man had not even taken an X-ray, I decided against him and just figured I would try to ride it out. I used a knee brace and ace-bandages, stayed away from over-working my knees and gradually the problem subsided and went away.

Two years back, my current G.P., who is a cardiologist and internist as well as a great believer in natural medicine, suggested that I begin regularly taking Glucosamin/Chondroitin, which is for the joints and since then I have had absolutely no problems with my knees. I have even tried slow jogging and it did not seem to bother them.

My ex-wife has been regularly taking 500 mg of Calcium in additional to her daily multivitamin/mineral supplements, to help stave off the onset of osteoporosis in women after menopause. I have read that too much Calcium for men (more than the system actually requires) can cause nasty deposits in your system, so I decided to take only 250 mg, with Magnesium, which can help keep bones strong and prevent muscle cramps.

I have, since my mid-twenties, always had elevated Cholesterol, but not to any serious degree. At one point, my Doctor recommended that I take one of the popular anti-Cholesterol drugs. After I read that one of the side effects of those drugs for some people could possibly be a problem with the liver, especially if you *drink regularly*. I quickly decided against it.

What I did try was a natural Cholesterol-inhibitor, called "Cholesterol Success" manufactured by TwinLab. Two tablets with breakfast and two with dinner, served to reduce my Cholesterol count by 25% within the first 60 days. Needless to say you have to watch your fat intake, but these supplements clearly seem to help.

Last but not least, like many people over sixty-five, I can remember what happened twenty years ago as though it was yesterday, but I can't remember what happened yesterday. So I decided to try the natural memory enhancer, Gingko Baloba.

My esteemed nutritionist, Lisa Cosman, has pointed out that Gingko has been suspected of elevating blood pressure levels in some people, so I took her advice and recently abandoned it.

I mattered little since I kept forgetting to take the damned tablet anyway.

The vitamins, minerals and supplements that I've just discussed are, of course, not going to be right for everyone, but they've worked for me. That's why I wanted to describe them in this chapter. For most people, a good multivitamin/mineral supplement will go a long way toward helping to maintain a healthy mind and body.

One final point; Let's talk briefly about fats and cholesterol. A regular exercise program, combined with an improved diet, can help to reduce your "bad" cholesterol and increase your "good" cholesterol.

Needless to say it's always in your best interest to keep your blood cholesterol down. A few paragraphs back, I mentioned "Cholesterol Success" a natural cholesterol blocker, which has no deleterious effects upon the liver. There are also a number of other natural cholesterol blockers which can also be quite effective.

But no matter what kind of a supplement you take or how much you exercise, you still need to watch your saturated fat intake. *Avoid any food that includes "partially hydrogenated oils" in its list of contents, even if the nutritional label claims zero grams of trans fats.* Many knowledgeable experts believe that "trans-fatty acids" are even worse for you than too much cholesterol.

There are various ways to keep the saturated fats and cholesterol intake down. I'm sure that you already are aware of the fact that the foods containing the highest content of saturated fats are real butter, real eggs, fatty meats, whole egg mayonnaise, whole milk or cream, real cheeses and rich desserts made with cream such as ice-cream and cheesecake.

Years ago your only choices were either real butter or margarine. Butter was loaded with saturated fat and cholesterol and margarine contained partially hydrogenated oils. Happily today there is another great choice. Margarine made with expeller-pressed oils. It is low in saturated fat, has no trans-fatty acids and it tastes like real butter.

There are two excellent substitutes for real eggs. You can either separate the whites from the yolk (egg whites are fat free), cook the whites for yourself and give the cooked yolks to the dog; or you can use a fat-free egg substitute like "Scramblers" or "Egg Beaters". They taste fine and make great scrambled eggs and omelets. You can even buy liquid egg whites in a container.

As for mayonnaise, you can get great tasting mayo made with expeller-pressed oils in most health food stores, or you can use low-fat mayo, which also has no trans-fatty acids.

Unless you're a baby, you simply do not need to drink whole milk. 1 or 2 percent reduced fat milk tastes great and skimmed milk nowadays is not like the seemingly watered down stuff you got years ago.

Cheeses now come in a variety of low-fat forms. Of course if you love cheese, it's real hard to find an acceptable cholesterol-free substitute, but the "veggie" cheeses are quite tasty. They come in American, Swiss, Cheddar, Mozzarella, Provolone, Pepper Jack and a host of other choices.

Apart from "veggie" cheeses, there are also a number of good-tasting fat free or low fat cheeses available in health food stores, which melt when heated.

Ice cream and frozen yogurt now are offered in fat-free and low-fat choices and most supermarkets now carry low-carb, low fat cheesecake.

As far as meats are concerned, simply trim off as much fat as you can before cooking. Turkey, white meat chicken and fish are lower in fats than red meats and they also afford you the psychological advantage of believing that you are eating light.

The point to remember, if you want to lower your blood cholesterol effectively you need to change your eating habits. Today, unlike when I was young, there are numerous wonderful low fat, cholesterol-free foods from which you can choose.

Eight

Now we start the dinner section of our diet. Here you get to increase your total number of selections to 2 ½ and also try some surprisingly delicious low-carb dishes and substitutes.

What about the dinner choices? I'm not going to repeat the choices I outlined for breakfast or luncheon. If you wish you can select *any* of those choices for dinner.

What I'm going to present to you now are some additional selections you might pick for dinner, which are more in line traditional meals. Later we'll get into some fairly exotic recipes designed to pique the proverbial palate.

You have a total of 2 1/2 choices, which should consist of one full choice and three half choices for your final meal of the day.

The first half choice should be a single slice of low-carb bread, Melba toast, or 2 saltine crackers, with butter or expeller pressed margarine. If you forego that you may use the ½ choice elsewhere.

Meat or fish is your second half choice. You can now enjoy up to 6 oz of any lean meat, including steak, chicken, lamb, pork or ham; as well as any type of seafood. Broil it, bake it, grill or fry it, as you wish, and use cooking oil sparingly. The spray-on cooking oils are preferable. If you like gravy, use a little on your meat, but buy the kind sold in 12 oz jars, or cans, which is low in carbs. They even have a fat-free version. The meat or fish counts as one-half choice, with nothing additional for gravy.

A few words here about George Forman's "Lean and Mean Grilling Machine". I just cannot say enough about this unit. Priced between $50 and $99, depending upon the size of the cooking surface; it grills even frozen meats relatively quickly, draining off fats as it cooks. It's also excellent for grilled veggies, tofu or eggplant as well as meat slices and veggies in low-carb wraps.

During the summer it doesn't heat up your kitchen like the oven nor does it let off any smoke in the grilling process. It's also quite easy to clean by removing the grilling plates and soaking them in hot soapy water for about 30 minutes.

The third half- choice can be veggies; a generous portion, if you wish. No corn, beets, stewed tomatoes, peas, baked beans or other high carb veggies. Soya beans are okay if you wish. You can dress up the veggies as you like, but watch any added carbs.

Grilling or broiling is desirable for many veggies, especially mushrooms, broccoli florets, cauliflower, yellow squash slices, cabbage chunks, peppers, eggplant and asparagus. Steamed vegetables are excellent as well, usually maintaining their crispness after cooking.

One of my favorite vegetables is a bunch of fresh spinach. Microwave it for about 40 to 60 seconds, or drop in boiling water for 7 to 10 seconds and drain. Splash on a small amount of soy sauce, sesame oil, sesame seeds and bit of course black pepper.

I also love fresh asparagus. Microwave or grill for about five minutes until cooked to your liking. Serve with salt and pepper and top with two spoonfuls of expeller pressed mayonnaise and they are absolutely superb.

If you want to substitute a generous-sized side salad for the veggies, that's fine. However, do not add croutons or nuts, except almond slivers. Keep the dressing low carb.

The only full choice, of your total 2 ½ is a pasta, rice or potato substitute.

Pasta is the easiest. Using organic, whole grain pasta, you can cook 1/8th of an eight oz package. Boil it with one tablespoon of olive oil and ½ tablespoon of salt. If you use low-carb pasta, you may increase the amount to ¼ of an eight oz package.

The best low-carb pasta that I have found is made by "Dreamfields". They make a penne or spaghetti which is the closest thing to regular pasta you will find. Even though the published carb count is higher, the body only absorbs 5 grams of carbs per serving. It cooks up soft and will satisfy any pasta craving you may be burdened with. The best place to find it is in your local health food store, but some supermarkets are also carrying the product. Should you not be able to obtain "Dreamfields" pastas, you can order them from their website, www17.netrition.com.

Shiratake is a relatively new pasta substitute, made from tofu, containing only 3 grams of carbs per serving. It is deliciously soft and palatable, sold either in fettuchini or spaghetti form. If not available in your local supermarket or Asian supermarket, check out the website at www.locarbu.com.

****

As a general reference tool, click on www.netrition.com for information on a virtual myriad of low carb food products.

****

For a rice substitute (Quasi-rice) you can grate or otherwise chop using an Osterizer, fresh cauliflower, peeled small white turnips, peeled yellow squash or very firm tofu, all of which yield a product almost the consistency of rice. Boil to desired softness, drain and serve.

For chopping I prefer the Osterizer (or a lower-priced generic brand). The unit isn't costly and is excellent for chopping onions, celery, cheeses, cooked meats, etc. If you don't want to invest in one, most department stores sell a very inexpensive manual chopper, which will also do the job, but not as well.

I like to add a mixture of a packet of instant broth to one oz of boiling water. You can also garnish the quasi-rice with chopped mushrooms, asparagus, broccoli, or slices of other veggies if you wish.

Optionally you may add 1/8th of a cup of Orzo pasta, which is the same size and consistency of long grain rice. Boil the Orzo, drain and add to cooked quasi rice. Mix well and serve as you would regular rice.

Last are potato substitutes, with which you can be very imaginative. For "Quasi French fries", cut "*super* firm" tofu (*found only in oriental food stores*) into French fried slices, preferably deep fry or pan-fry until brown. Add a sprinkle of garlic and onion powder if you wish. You can also use "extra firm" tofu found in the super markets, but it's not quite as good for quasi fries, as the *super* firm oriental store tofu. In addition, regular tofu must be <u>fully drained</u> and, after cutting, patted firmly against a few layers of paper towels to remove any water.

You can also French fry fresh cauliflower florets or sliced small white turnips. Just add oil to a pan and fry or deep-fry until partially brown.

For quasi-mashed potatoes you start with 4 to 6 oz of frozen cauliflower florets, which is a wonderful substitute, and microwave or boil until soft. Then mash as you would potatoes, or mix in the Osterizer, until the consistency is just like mashed potatoes. You can add a little salt and butter and a very small amount of milk or half and half. Instead of milk, if you wish, you can instead add a few tablespoons of expeller-pressed sour cream and some grated Parmesan cheese for a very nice taste. Serve garnished with parsley or gravy, if you wish. A touch of onion and garlic powder added to the mashed cauliflower also adds a nice touch. Alternatively, one tablespoon of horseradish added to the mix, imparts an interesting tangy flavor.

To carry that a bit further and make quasi-baked potatoes, shape a few small pieces of aluminum foil wrap so that they're the size and shape of a half baked-potato skin. Fill with the quasi potatoes and sprinkle with chives. Broil for a few minutes and serve plain or topped with brown gravy, or shredded low fat cheddar cheese. If plain, you can serve with light expeller-pressed sour cream. You may also sprinkle on cheese powder instead of sour cream or cheddar cheese. You will recall, that is the powdered cheese found in a box of macaroni and cheese.

You may also select Dreamfields or whole grain noodles as your *complete* dinner meal. Take two oz of uncooked whole grain noodles (1/4 of an 8 oz box) or four oz of Dreamfields noodles, and add a half-tablespoon of salt and a tablespoon of olive oil to the water to give it a nice taste. Boil the noodles until tender.

Serve your choice of noodles with one or two tablespoons of olive oil and a tablespoon of cider vinegar and sprinkle with parmesan cheese (or sesame oil and a tablespoon of rice vinegar and no parmesan cheese).

As another dressing, you may also use lobster or clam sauce or marinara sauce. If you like, you can add up to five pieces of cooked shrimp or (to the Marinara sauce) three turkey meatballs, or one sausage link, without increasing the total selection count. You may also have a small side salad and one slice of low-carb bread.

If you like tofu or eggplant, cut soft tofu into ¾ inch cubes, or uncooked eggplant into slices into ¼ inch slices, and broil or grill either or both for a few minutes, with any combination of the following; fresh mushrooms, onions, carrot slices, broccoli and a few small cuts of cabbage. Before broiling, or grilling, garnish with (*either*) General Tso's sauce, Chinese marinade, teriyaki or peanut sauce, or simply brown gravy. The gravy sold in jars or cans is fairly low in carbs.

Broiled artichoke hearts, either frozen or canned, sprayed with oil are very good as a sumptuous change. Additionally broiled or grilled slices of yellow squash garnished with teriyaki sauce are quite delicious.

Quasi Rice

Ingredients:

For quasi rice, use two cups of either fresh white cauliflower florets, or peeled white turnips, or peeled yellow squash, or semi-firm tofu.

Also, optionally, you may add 1/8th cup of Orzo pasta uncooked (which is the same size as long grain rice).

Directions:

Grate or chop the cauliflower, turnips or squash with an Osterizer, manual chopper or cheese grater, until the consistency is similar to rice.

Boil to desired tenderness

Boil the 1/8th cup of Orzo pasta, drain and add to the quasi rice.

Quasi Mashed Potatoes

Ingredients:

Frozen cauliflower florets 4 to 6 oz

½ oz of whole milk or low fat expeller-pressed sour cream 2 tablespoons

Butter or expeller-pressed margarine, 1 tablespoon

Horseradish, 1 teaspoon (optional)

Parmesan cheese (optional)

Directions:

Boil or microwave the frozen cauliflower florets until soft as boiled potatoes; drain

Mash as you would potatoes, adding salt and butter. I prefer to use the Osterizer instead of mashing.

Add a small amount of whole milk or expeller-pressed sour cream if you wish. A teaspoon or tablespoon of horseradish added to the quasi mix imparts a lovely tangy taste. Alternatively, some added grated Parmesan cheese lovely.

Garnish with parsley or brown gravy

Quasi Baked Potatoes

Ingredients:

Quasi Mashed Potatoes

Aluminum foil shaped like a half-baked potato skin

Chives, expeller-pressed sour cream, gravy or shredded cheddar cheese

Directions:

Place the quasi-mashed potatoes into the aluminum foil pockets.

Broil at 450 for about seven minutes

If you use the shredded cheddar cheese, sprinkle it on before broiling.

If you do not use the cheese, cover the quasi-mashed potatoes with chives, expeller-pressed sour cream or gravy.

Nine

Let's discuss drinking alcoholic beverages.

I think you know by now that for as many of my mature years as I can recall, I've been routinely consuming three to four full-bodied beers before dinner and even substituting a few glasses of wine for a few of the beers (e.g. one or two wines for one or two of the beers).

I know that full-bodied beers add a significant amount of carbs to my daily total, but it's the one pleasure I haven't deprived myself of while following this diet. I also believe that had I embarked upon this diet and also attempted to quit drinking at the same time, I wouldn't have been successful. But that's me and not necessarily for you; different strokes.

Again, if you don't drink, or if you drink abstemiously, that's fine. If you do drink beer and would like to try and keep the carbs low, there are a few things that you can do to cut them.

First, you can drink light beer instead of full-bodied. Most light beers today are great tasting, very low in carbs and have about the same alcoholic content as regular beers.

Yes, you still get the buzz.

An easy way to make the transition is to start by substituting your first beer of the evening with a light beer. The following night substitute the first two beers with light. Then three, four, etc. until you're drinking only light beers.

I did it a number of years back and it worked fine. After a week or ten days I was truly enjoying the light beers and not missing the full-bodied beers. It was working fine, until one of the holidays when I was entertaining my close family and a few other relatives. I was feeling so good that I asked myself,.....

'So what's the big deal if I have a few regular beers today? I can pick up my light beer regimen tomorrow.'

Not true for this camper.

I went right back to drinking full-bodied beers.

It was just like the few times I tried to decaffeinate.

I was doing okay on decaffeinated coffee. I got past the withdrawal and found that I wasn't feeling tired in the mornings or late afternoon, when I normally have my caffeine jolts. As a matter of fact, my level of energy was steadier without regular coffee.

So one afternoon, I thought,....

'What the heck? One cup of real coffee won't kill me.'

The enormous buzz that I felt after that single cup was almost like taking Benzedrine diet pills years ago. I felt renewed, rejuvenated, highly invigorated. Ready to lick the world.

Of course I had blown it and was back on regular coffee.

You can also reduce your intake of full-bodied beers by starting the evening with two bottles of non-alcoholic beer, then moving to regulars. You will find after four beers, two non-alcoholic and two regulars, that you may have reached your fill of beers for the night.

You can also cut the carbs and alcohol in wine by taking a one liter bottle of wine and diluting it with one part water or seltzer (20%), to four parts wine. If you serve it *ice cold*, chilled for a while in the freezer, it's not bad at all.

You might try a wine Spritzer by adding 7 oz of seltzer, diet ginger ale, or any other diet soda, two oz of wine. Or try 7 oz of tonic to two oz of wine. In any of these three drinks, serve in a tall glass with ice cubs.

You can also enjoy a delicious Bloody Mary by adding two oz of dry wine (or one oz of vodka), to 7 oz of low-carb vegetable juice cocktail (see recipe in Chapter Four), then handily spicing it up with a few dashes of Worsteshire and Tabasco sauces.

The previous four paragraphs are merely suggestions, based upon my own experience that you may wish to try.

From a personal standpoint, I've lost my weight and managed to maintain the lower weight despite continuing to drink full-bodied beers and full strength wine.

What the hell, life is too damned short.

Ten

Now, let's look at some tasty dinner dishes, which will add more variety and spice to your menu. Remember that the recipes for these selections are all shown at the end of the chapter and there's also an alphabetical index to all recipes at the end of the book.

How about Japanese Negemaki, or Tempura; steak with cognac sauce; honey glazed chicken?

Perhaps you might like some chicken with rice? Or beef with broccoli and rice? Or Pepper steak with rice?

Okay, but we can't eat *real* rice on this diet can we? All of these dishes are great with the quasi-rice shown in Chapter Eight. Chicken with rice is fairly simple; add chunks of cooked white meat chicken to the quasi-rice and pour on some condensed broth. I use one packet of instant chicken or beef broth to one oz of boiling water. Toss in cooked mushrooms or any veggie you like and you've got a great chicken and rice substitute dish. You might like to add a small amount of butter or margarine with expeller pressed oils. *Butter Buds* are also great on quasi-rice.

Japanese Negemaki, Tempura and Teriyaki dishes make great low-carb entrees. They are all deceptively easy to prepare. For Negemaki, cut some fresh scallions into ¾ inch pieces, wrap about 6 pieces in a one inch thin-sliced strip of flank steak; place 6 to 8 of the wrapped Negemaki in a baking dish; add equal amounts of Soy Sauce, wine and lemon juice; then a small amount of sweetener to soften the tang of the lemon and Soy Sauce. Bake at 475 for 6 minutes, then broil for an additional four minutes, without turning.

Tempura is made by adding water to Tempura powder (available in most oriental food stores), until the mixture forms a creamy texture. Dip shrimps; or small pieces of fish, chicken, pork, lamb or beef into the mixture to coat, then deep fry for a few minutes until crispy brown. You can also dip and fry, eggplant, mushrooms, carrots, squash, zucchini, green or red bell pepper slices, virtually any veggie. You must make the powder/water mixture thick enough so that it will coat the pieces to be deep fried, but try to keep it thin, since the thinner the mix the lower the carb count.

Teriyaki is a breeze. Coat salmon, chicken breasts, or steak with Teriyaki sauce or glaze (which has a thicker consistency); then broil or grill until done to your taste. You can always add some additional Teriyaki sauce to use over veggies or quasi-rice. Be certain to cross-cut the steak into thin slices before adding the sauce.

For Steak with cognac sauce, use cognac and your favorite barbecue sauce, plus olive oil, garlic powder, cracked pepper, beef bullion, horseradish and flour.

Rub olive oil over steaks and sprinkle on cracked pepper and minced garlic.

In a bowl; to 1/3 cup of water, add 2 packets of beef bullion, 1 teaspoon of horseradish, 1 tablespoon of flour and bring to a boil; add ½ cup of cognac and ¼ cup of barbecue sauce, simmer and stir until the mix thickens slightly.

Grill, broil or fry the steaks as you prefer.

Pour the cognac mix over the sizzling hot steaks.

Serve with grilled veggies, cooked spinach; or quasi-baked potatoes

Honey glazed chicken is made by adding 2-3 tablespoon of Dijon mustard to ¼ cup of honey, 1 packet of sweetener and a teaspoon of lemon juice. Generously garnish chicken breasts, wings or thighs; and broil, grill or bake. Serve with grilled veggies; cooked spinach or quasi-baked potatoes.

Here, for you Italian food lovers, are a few great low-carb dishes. By the way, in any recipe where I recommend covering the contents with a layer of mozzarella, I usually suggest that you cover the cheese with a thin spray coating of olive oil; the commercial olive oil spray available in supermarkets. This is a completely optional step, depending on how dry or moist you like your melted mozzarella cheese.

Do you like ziti? Boil one oz of whole grain ziti or penne noodles with a bit of olive oil and salt in the water, drain and put into a baking dish with fresh sliced mushroom and zucchini. Cover with 4 – 6 oz of marinara sauce, or any of your favorite Italian sauces.

I like to make my own sauce, by combining a small can of tomato past with a 16 oz can of Del Monte's Italian Stewed Tomatoes. I add ½ tspn of garlic powder and 1/3rd cup of water. Break up the tomatoes with a fork to achieve a better consistency.

Sprinkle on a layer of three or four oz of low fat shredded mozzarella cheese. Spray a thin coat of olive oil over the cheese and bake at 450 for about 20 minutes, until the cheese is brown and crispy.

As an option, you can add two tablespoons of low-fat Ricotta cheese (or fat-free cottage cheese) to the noodles, before adding the sauce.

Serve one slice of low-carb bread and a small side salad.

Baked eggplant is a wonderful Italian dish. In a baking dish, place fresh ¼ inch eggplant slices. Bake them alone at 350 for twenty minutes and drain off any liquid; or else grill the eggplant slices for 30 to 45 seconds. Add fresh mushrooms, sliced black olives, chopped onions and a small amount of sliced zucchini. Sprinkle on a little Parmesan cheese and cover with a layer of Marinara or your favorite sauce. Place a layer of shredded low-fat mozzarella cheese on top, spray on a thin layer of olive oil and bake at 350 for about 15 minutes or until the cheese is crispy brown. A bit of provolone cheese mixed with the mozzarella imparts a nice nutty taste.

I love Calzone. It's easy to make a low-carb version. Mix four oz of Ricotta or fat-free cottage cheese, with four oz of shredded low fat mozzarella cheese, ¼ of a thin sliced green pepper and some chopped onions or scallions. Place the mix in two large low-carb wraps; lay thin strips of cooked sausage sliced lengthwise, or a small amount of ham strips, on top of the mixture. Close up the wraps and bake at 350 for 15 minutes.

I must confess that I'm a take-out Chinese food freak. I have always loved Lo Mein, fried jumbo shrimps, egg rolls, fried rice and the like. The problem is that most of these foods are very high in carbs, due to the fact that they are traditionally served with white rice or noodles.

Here are a few tasty low-carb substitutes for Chinese take out food.

For beef with broccoli, take 6 oz of chuck steak and boil in 8 to 10 oz of water in a covered pot with three or four packets of instant beef broth, or a generous dash of Gravy Master, for about an hour, until it's virtually falling apart with tenderness. It should be very soft in about an hour.

Cut the cooked meat into thin slices and add cooked broccoli florets, a bit of chopped onion, sliced mushrooms and a small amount of thin-sliced julienne-style carrots. Put the whole mixture into brown gravy, heat until the mushrooms are cooked and serve alone or over your rice substitute. You can substitute chunks of chicken, pork or shrimp for the beef if you wish.

Pepper steak is easy as well. After preparing your beef as above, remove it and place on the side. In a lightly oiled skillet, sauté chopped onions, green pepper and mushrooms. Add a jar of brown gravy, with three to four tablespoons of Chinese Marinade or General Tso's sauce if you have it; if not the brown gravy alone is just fine. Add the cooked meat, heat and serve alone or over your rice substitute.

Let's take the fried jumbo shrimps, which if you will note, are normally covered with a layer of breadcrumbs that is a least ¼ inch in thickness. Instead take ¾ of cup of flour, which makes a significantly thinner coating than regular breadcrumbs. Mix with water enough water so that it adopts a thin gravy-like consistency. Dip large *pre-cooked frozen jumbo shrimps* into the mix and then deep-fry them for about a half-to-one minute or until golden brown.

The next dish is Lo-Mein, which consists of thin spaghetti noodles, with varieties of vegetables, mixed with a gravy-like sauce and either served alone or with added shrimp, beef, pork or chicken. First boil ½ oz of whole grain spaghetti noodles, drain and put aside. Add a small amount of oil to a large skillet. Sautee fresh mushrooms, sliced onions or scallions, a small amount of julienne-style carrots and chopped cabbage. You can also add a bit of thin sliced celery if you wish. If you wish to add some thin-sliced extra-firm tofu, reduce the amount of noodles by the amount of tofu that you use.

When the mixture is well sautéed, add a small amount of chopped green pepper and a can of drained bean sprouts (available in any regular supermarket in the oriental food section). Finally add your cooked noodles, a half jar of brown beef gravy (and a few optional tablespoons of General Tso's sauce, Chinese Marinade, or peanut sauce). Mix it well; add a little soy sauce and you have a great low-carb Lo-Mein. You can serve it alone or with added cooked shrimp, or small slices of cooked beef, pork or chicken.

I could go on forever.

For egg rolls, take the exact same mixture as for Lo-Mein, without *the noodles, gravy, or sauce,* mix it up and fill a few low-carb wraps. Roll up the wraps to close in the mixture and deep fry or bake in the oven or toaster oven until the wraps are slightly brown. Again, if you like, you can add a small amount of cooked shrimp, beef, pork or chicken to the egg roll.

Fried quasi-rice is easy as well. Sautee fresh mushrooms, onions, celery and julienne-style carrots. Then add a small amount of chopped green and red peppers, a half-cup of scrambled fat free eggs. Put that aside and take your cooked quasi-rice and stir-fry for a few minutes in a skillet, using Canola oil, then toss with the sautéed mixture and a small amount of soy sauce.

As an oriental salad, you can take a small amount of chopped lettuce and top it with a few tablespoons of Kim Chee. Most health food stores carry a mild version, if the typical Korean Kim Chee is too spicy for you.

If you love the crispy Chinese dry noodles that traditionally come with Chinese soup or Chow Mein, you can take a low-carb wrap, spray it with a thin coating of oil and cut it up into small pieces resembling the Chinese noodles. Spread them onto a sheet of aluminum foil and bake in a toaster oven until brown and crispy.

For egg drop soup, you can start with chicken broth and bring it to a boil. Slowly drop in uncooked eggs or egg whites, a half-teaspoon at a time, stirring quickly as raw eggs or egg whites hit the boiling broth.

You can make very delicious spare ribs by broiling pork ribs garnished with a thin coating of Sweet and Sour sauce. This is equal to one choice. A lower-carb alternative to the Sweet and Sour sauce is; 2 oz of sugar-free orange marmalade, with 2 oz of sugar-free strawberry jam, 2 teaspoons of spicy or hot mustard and 1 teaspoon of vinegar.

All of the above should serve to satisfy most Chinese take-out lovers and still keep the carbs very low.

In a previous chapter we covered a variety of nice low-carb dishes that you can have for lunch. Needless to say, you can partake of any of them for dinner as well.

That's it for dinner. There's a listing all of all of your dinner choices in the last few pages of the book. After the following recipes we'll move on to desserts and snacks.

Negemaki

Ingredients:

Flank steak 6 oz

6 Scallions

Lemon Juice

White wine

Sweetener

Directions:

Slice the raw flank steak against the grain into thin slices each about 6 inches long

Wash and cut scallions into ¾ inch pieces

Form six pieces of scallion standing on edge, into a round cluster and

Wrap one slice of flank steak about the scallions; place into a baking dish – repeat with the rest of the scallions and steak slices.

Pour in equal parts soy sauce, wine and lemon juice to cover one half of the Negemaki – add a small amount of sweetener to cut the tartness

Bake 4 – 6 minutes then broil for an additional 4 minutes. Serve with quasi rice, if desired

Tempura

Ingredients:

Shrimp, Beef, Chicken, Salmon or Pork

Canola oil

Tempura powder

Fresh vegetables, if desired -- florets of broccoli; cauliflower; sliced carrots; sliced mushrooms; sliced eggplant; onions; squash; green or red bell peppers

Directions:

Mix tempura powder and water in a large bowl to create a thin creamy consistency; if you are also going to cook the vegetables place ½ of the mixture aside. Cut the shrimp, salmon, or meat into bite-sized pieces and dip the pieces into the Tempura mix.

Deep fry the fish or meat until brown and crispy. If you are also cooking vegetables, dip the fresh vegetables into the other half of the Tempura mixture. Deep fry the vegetables a very short time.

Teriyaki

Ingredients:

Steak, chicken, pork, salmon, tuna or shrimp
Teriyaki sauce or glaze

Directions:

Place meat or fish in baking pan, cover liberally with Teriyaki sauce and broil.

Steak With Cognac

Ingredients:

4 Filet Mignon Steaks

½ Cup of Cognac

¼ Cup of Barbeque sauce

Olive oil

Cracked Pepper and minced garlic

2 Packets of Beef bullion

1 teaspoon of Horseradish

1 tablespoon of flour

Directions:

In a skillet, combine 1/3 cup water, 2 packets of beef broth, 1 teaspoon of horseradish, and 1 tablespoon of flour and bring to a boil. Add ½ cup of cognac and ¼ cup of barbeque sauce, simmer and stir until the mix thickens.

Rub olive oil and cracked pepper over the filet mignon steaks and then lightly sprinkle on some minced garlic. Broil or grill steaks to your liking.

Slice cooked filet mignon into thin slices and pour cognac sauce on top.

Serve with grilled veggies or quasi baked potatoes.

Steak Balsamic

Ingredients:

4 Filet Mignon Steaks

Lemon juice

Horseradish

Sweetener

Balsamic vinegar

Dijon Mustard

Directions:

Mix ¼ cup of balsamic vinegar with 1 tablespoon of Dijon Mustard, 2 teaspoons of lemon juice, 2 teaspoons horseradish and a packet of sweetener.

Marinade 4 Filet Mignon Steaks or 2 Rib Steaks for 15 minutes in the mixed balsamic sauce then broil the steak liberally garnished in sauce.

Serve with grilled veggies; cooked spinach; or quasi-baked potatoes

Honey Mustard Glazed Chicken

Directions:

Mix ¼ cup of honey with 2 – 3 tablespoons of Dijon mustard and one tea of lemon juice and 1 packet of sweetener

Coat chicken wings, thighs or breast liberally with mixture

Grill or Broil and serve with grilled veggies; cooked spinach; or Quasi-rice.

Ziti -_Baked

Ingredients

Whole grain Ziti or Penne noodles – 1 oz

Marinara sauce or any of your favorite spaghetti sauces - 4 to 6 oz

Sliced fresh mushrooms and sliced zucchini

Shredded low fat Mozzarella cheese – 4 to 6 oz

Olive oil spray

Olive oil and salt

(Optionally) 2 tablespoons of Ricotta or fat free cottage cheese.

Directions:

Boil noodles until soft (in water with salt and small amount olive oil) drain and cool.

Mix the noodles in a baking dish with ¼ of the sauce, the sliced mushrooms and zucchini (and optionally, the Ricotta or Cottage cheese).

Sprinkle remaining sauce over noodles

Cover with a layer of shredded mozzarella cheese

Spray a thin coat of olive oil over the cheese

Bake @ 425, until the cheese is brown and crispy

Baked Eggplant Parmigiana

Ingredients:

Fresh eggplant, sliced as desired

Fresh mushrooms, black olives, onions and zucchini

Parmesan cheese (2 tablespoons)

Spaghetti sauce

Shredded low fat mozzarella cheese - 4 to 6 oz

Olive oil spray

Directions:

Bake the eggplant slices at 350 for twenty minutes and drain off any liquid; or grill for 30 to 45 seconds

Slice the mushrooms, zucchini, onions and black olives; mix with the eggplant and Parmesan cheese in a baking dish (the mixture should be 2/3rds eggplant to 1/3 of the rest)

Cover with a generous layer of spaghetti sauce

Cover with the shredded mozzarella cheese

Spray a light coating of olive oil and bake @ 425 until cheese is melted and crisp

Roger's Special "Del Monte" Italian Sauce

Directions:

One 6 oz can of tomato paste and one 16 oz can of Del Monte Italian Stewed Tomatoes.

1/3 cup water and ½ tspn garlic powder

Combine all ingredients in a sauce pan. Crush tomatoes slightly with a fork and heat, stirring with a spoon.

Calzone

Ingredients:

Ricotta or fat free cottage cheese - 4 oz

Shredded low fat mozzarella cheese - 4 oz

¼ green pepper

one small onion or a few scallions

1 pre-cooked Italian sausage or slice of ham

2 large low carb wraps

Directions:

Cut the green pepper into thin slices.

Chop the onions or scallions

Mix with the Ricotta or cottage cheese and mozzarella cheese

Place 1/2 of the mixture in each low carb wrap.

Slice the sausage or ham lengthwise into long thin pieces and lay the pieces over the cheese mixture

Close up the wraps

Using a thin sheet of aluminum foil, wrap up each Calzone and bake @ 350 for 15 minutes

Chicken with Rice (Quasi)

Ingredients:

Quasi rice ingredients

Chunks of pre-cooked white meat chicken

Fresh mushrooms

½ cup of broccoli florets or asparagus

2 packets of chicken broth

1 teaspoon of honey

Directions:

Prepare Quasi rice as in the Quasi rice recipe.

Mix 2 packets of chicken broth with ½ cup of water and 1 tspn. honey.

Chop broccoli or asparagus to smaller pieces and blanche them

Mix with quasi rice

Lay on chicken slices

Pour chicken broth over everything

Beef* and Broccoli

Ingredients:

Chuck steak; 6 to 8 oz

2 cups of broccoli florets

Gravy Master

1 medium onion and sliced fresh mushrooms

Julienne style carrots; $1/3^{rd}$ cup

Brown Gravy, mixed with 3 to 4 tablespoons of Chinese Marinade

Quasi rice ingredients

Directions:

Prepare Quasi rice as in Quasi Rice recipe

Boil the chuck steak for about an hour in water with 4 tablespoons of Gravy Master, until the meat is literally falling apart. Cut into thin slices.

Slice the mushrooms and onion.

Blanche the broccoli, mushrooms, onion and carrots. Mix with the Brown Gravy and Chinese Marinade.

Lay the beef slices over the quasi rice.

Cover with the Gravy and blanched vegetables.

* You may substitute chicken, pork, or shrimps for the chuck steak, but do not cook as long as you would the beef.

Pepper Steak

Ingredients:

Chuck steak; 8 to 10 oz

One medium sized green pepper and one small onion

Fresh mushrooms

Brown gravy mixed with 2 tablespoons Chinese Marinade or General Tso's sauce

Directions:

Prepare steak as in Beef with Broccoli recipe

Slice onions, peppers and mushrooms and Sautee in a small amount of oil

Prepare Quasi Rice as in previous recipes

Lay sautéed vegetables over quasi rice

Lay slices of steak over vegetables and rice

Cover with Brown Gravy mixed with 2 tablespoons Chinese Marinade or General Tso's sauce

Fried Jumbo Shrimps

Ingredients:

Frozen pre-cooked shrimps

Canola oil 16 oz

¾ cup of flour

Directions:

Mix 1 cup of the flour with water (about 1/5th of a cup), to achieve the consistency of a creamy soup.

Dip the frozen shrimp in the mix

Bring oil to a boil and deep fry shrimps for 15 – 30 seconds until brown and crispy.

Lo-Mein

Ingredients:

2 oz of whole grain spaghetti noodles, or Dreamfields low carb noodles or one package of Shiratake noodles.

Fresh mushrooms, celery, onions or scallions, julienne-style carrots (1/8th cup), green pepper

1/5th of a head of chopped cabbage

1 can drained bean sprouts

Brown gravy with 3 to 4 tablespoons of Chinese Marinade or General Tso's sauce, or peanut sauce

Directions:

Boil the noodles until soft, drain and put aside

Slice the mushrooms, onions or scallions and green pepper

Slice the celery to very thin slices

Chop the cabbage and Sautee with the mushrooms, onions, green pepper, celery, julienne carrots and drained bean sprouts

Add the cooked noodles

Add a half jar of the brown gravy mixed with Chinese Marinade or the peanut, or General Tso's sauce

Serve alone or with added shrimp, pork, beef or chicken

Egg Rolls

Ingredients:

Use the same ingredients as for Lo-Mein, except without the noodles and gravy

Plus

2 – 3 low carb wraps

Olive oil spray

Directions:

Sautee mix as for Lo-Mein

Fill the low carb wraps and roll up to close in the mixture

Deep Fry, about one minute, until golden brown or

Bake at 250 until wraps are slightly brown.

You can also add chunks of shrimp, chicken, beef or pork

Quasi Fried Rice

Ingredients:

Prepare Quasi Rice per recipe (including boiling to desired softness) and drain thoroughly

Fresh mushrooms

1 small to medium onion

¼ green pepper

¼ red pepper

½ cup cooked scrambled eggs

1/8 cup julienne-style carrots

Soy Sauce

Directions:

Fry the prepared quasi-rice for 2 minutes in a skillet under a high-flame, skillet, tossing frequently.

Chop vegetables and Sautee with pre-scrambled eggs

Toss everything and add small amount of soy sauce.

Egg Drop Soup

Ingredients:

Four whole eggs

Salt

4 cups of Chicken Broth

Directions:

Use either whole uncooked eggs, or else separate the raw egg whites from the yolks and use only the whites (for less cholesterol)

If you use whole eggs, mix with a fork

Bring the broth to a high boil

Drop in the uncooked egg whites or whole eggs ½ teaspoon at a time, stirring quickly when eggs hit the boiling broth

Add salt to taste

SPECIALTY RECIPES
FOR GOURMETS,
FOR THOSE WHO FANCY THEMSELVES
GOURMETS,
AND FOR THOSE WHO HAVEN'T A CLUE

Mushroom Pork Chops

Ingredients:

4 Boneless Chops

Salt and Pepper (1/4 teaspoon combined)

1 cup chopped mushrooms

½ red bell pepper, chopped

1 can of Cream of Mushroom soup

½ cup of Expeller-pressed sour cream

Directions:

Slice chops flatways into 2 thinner flat pieces (e.g.: if your chop is 1 inch thick, you should end up with two slices, each ½ inch in thickness)

Mix all other ingredients in a saucepan and heat until soup is fully liquid. Spoon the mixture over one chop slice and place the second slice on top, sandwich style. Spoon the mix over the top. Secure with toothpicks.

Bake for 6 to 7 minutes at 450, then broil for an additional 2-3 minutes.

Marsala Chicken

Ingredients:

Thin sliced chicken breasts - 1 lb.

½ cup of Marsala wine

6 – 8 fresh mushrooms - sliced

3 tablespoons of Wondra flour

2 tablespoons of expeller pressed margarine

Directions:

Melt margarine

Lay chicken and mushrooms in a pan which has been lightly sprayed with oil

Pour over melted margarine and Marsala wine

Sprinkle flour over meat

Bake at 450 for 7 minutes (do not turn meat)

Spoon sauce over meat

Broil for an additional 3 minutes

Add salt to taste

Serve with grilled veggies

Stuffed Skirt Steak

Ingredients:

1 Pound of Skirt Steak

10 oz chopped frozen spinach

2 tablespoons Parmesan cheese

3 oz chopped low fat Monterey Jack cheese

¼ red bell pepper chopped

Directions:

Mix spinach, cheeses and pepper

Spoon the mix atop a slice of skirt steak

Roll each steak and secure with tooth picks

Bake at 500 for 7 minutes

Broil for an additional 3 minutes

Serve with grilled veggies

Montreal Skirt Steak

Ingredients:

1 lb. Skirt Steak

2 fresh limes

Garlic Powder

Powdered Thyme

Powdered Steak Seasoning

Directions:

Rub lime juice over entire steaks

Lay steaks in a broiling pan

Sprinkle on Garlic powder, Powdered Thyme and Steak seasoning

Broil 2 minutes

Turn steaks and sprinkle on Garlic powder, Powdered Thyme and Steak seasoning

Broil an additional 2 to 3 minutes

Serve with grilled veggies

Rib-Eye Stroganoff

Ingredients:

2 thick cut rib-eye steaks

1 teaspoons of each of the following: Rosemary, Powdered Thyme, Parsley, minced garlic, cracked pepper and Olive oil

2 teaspoons of Dijon Mustard

2 teaspoons of expeller pressed mayonnaise

½ cup of Expeller-pressed sour cream

Directions:

Mix spices

Rub oil over steaks

Rub spice mixture over oiled steaks

Broil steaks and slice thinly

For the sauce, stir 2 teaspoons Dijon Mustard with, the mayonnaise and expeller-pressed sour cream

Heat to a simmer

Spoon over steak slices

Serve with grilled veggies

Spinach/Broccoli Omelet With Monterey Jack

Ingredients:

1 cup fat free egg substitute

The whites of 2 eggs or ¼ cup of liquid egg whites

Dash of salt and pepper

½ cup of shredded low fat Monterey jack or Cheddar cheese

1 tablespoon finely chopped onions

1 cup fresh spinach leaves or

½ cup chopped broccoli

Directions:

Spray a large skillet with cooking oil spray

Heat well

Mix egg substitute with egg whites, onions, salt, pepper and pour into skillet

Cover skillet and cook on low flame until firm

Sprinkle over *half* of the eggs, the shredded cheese and the spinach leaves or chopped broccoli

With a spatula, carefully flip the uncovered half of the omelet over the half which has been covered with cheese and vegetables

Cook over low flame for a minute --- turn over the entire omelet and cook for two additional minutes

Shrimp/Crabmeat Asparagus

Ingredients:

12 fresh asparagus spears

Juice of one lime

¼ teaspoon of salt

2 tablespoons of expeller pressed margarine

9 cooked frozen jumbo shrimp

Frozen artificial crabmeat – 9 small chunks

3 tablespoons of mayonnaise

6 fresh mushrooms – sliced

Directions:

Cut asparagus spears in half and place in an oil sprayed baking dish

Lay in mushroom slices, shrimps and crabmeat

Bake at 450 for 10 -12 minutes - Place in a serving dish

Melt margarine, mix with the mayonnaise, lime juice and salt

Spoon over the baked asparagus, shrimp, crabmeat and mushrooms

Serve alone or over whole grain spaghetti noodles or quasi-rice

Seafood Supreme

Ingredients:

Fresh Calamari   4 - 6 pieces

Fresh Scallops   4 – 6 pieces

Frozen Artificial Crabmeat   4 - 6 chunks

Frozen pre-cooked jumbo shrimps   4 – 6 pieces

Liquid egg whites

Flour

Canola Oil

Tartar Sauce

Seafood Cocktail Sauce

Directions:

Dip all shellfish pieces into liquid egg whites

Roll pieces in a dish flour

Deep fry or pan fry, allowing fresh Calamari and Scallops to cook about 90 seconds before adding frozen shrimp and crabmeat pieces to oil.

Accompany with a small bowl of Tartar Sauce and one of Seafood Cocktail Sauce. Serve with grilled veggies.

Fried Lemon Chicken

Ingredients:

Chicken Thighs

Lemon Juice

Salt & Pepper

Flour

Canola Oil

Directions:

Marinade Chicken thighs in Lemon juice for ½ hour.

Add cold water to 1 cup of flour to form a thin creamy mix.

Lightly salt & pepper chicken thighs

Dip pieces into flour cream mix

Deep fry

Note: This is a much lower carb dish than standard fried chicken, which is either done with breadcrumbs or a lot of flour. Remember the thinner the flour/water mix, the less carbs; but if it is too thin, the receipt suffers.

Crispy Fried Chicken

You can also fry any kind of chicken (*without the lemon marinade*) using the above directions.

Lime Steak

Ingredients:

1 lb. of Skirt Steak or Filet Mignon

Cumin powder

Powdered Steak Seasoning

Juice of 3 Limes or 1/3 cup of reconstituted Lime Juice

Directions:

Marinade Steaks in lime juice for 1 hour

Sprinkle lightly with powdered Steak Seasoning

And liberally with Cumin powder

Broil or grill steaks

Port Rib-Eye Steak

Ingredients:

3 Thick Cut Rib-eye steaks

Black coarsely ground pepper

8 medium uncut fresh mushrooms

2 medium chopped onions

4 sliced black olives

½ red bell pepper cut into ¼ inch slices

2 teaspoons of barbecue sauce

1 packet of powdered beef broth

2 tablespoons of Port wine

1 tablespoon of Olive oil

2 tablespoons of expeller-pressed margarine

Directions

In a skillet, sauté mushrooms, olives, bell peppers, onions, barbecue sauce, in margarine - stir in Port wine, beef broth and 1/8 cup of water – Boil & simmer to thicken sauce

Rub uncooked steaks with oil and black pepper - Grill or broil

Slice broiled steaks into thin slices

Serve sliced steaks layered over grilled veggies

Generously cover with the Port sauce

Juicy Superior Montreal Steaks

Ingredients:

Thick cut Rib-eye, Strip or Porterhouse steaks

Liquid smoke (available in supermarkets)

Chef Paul Prudhomme's "Blackened Steak Magic" seasoning

Garlic Powder, lemon juice and 1 packet sweetener

Dash of Tabasco sauce

1 tablespoon of soy sauce and 1 tablespoon of olive oil

Directions:

Marinade the steaks one hour in a mixture of 1/2 cup of Lemon Juice, 1 tablespoon of soy sauce and 1 packet of sweetener - blot with paper towels before frying

Heat a large covered skillet over a high flame until very, very hot

Drop in steaks, sprinkle on liquid smoke and cover immediately

After one-half minute, sprinkle on powdered "Blackened Steak Magic" seasoning, garlic powder and a dash of Tabasco.

Turn steaks over; add 1 tablespoon of olive oil to pan – cover and continue to fry on high flame for 3 minutes

Sprinkle on more liquid smoke – "Blackened Steak Magic" seasoning and garlic powder. Turn steaks - cover and cook on high flame

After 1 - 2 minutes remove 1 steak and cut into it to ensure that the center is still very pink. Continue to fry until outside is darkened to your satisfaction.

Orange Pork Chops

Ingredients:

Sugar-free Orange Marmalade

Dijon Mustard

Orange Juice

Coarse black pepper

Directions:

Mix ½ cup of Orange Marmalade with 2 tablespoons of orange juice and 3 tablespoons of Dijon Mustard

Liberally garnish pork chops with Orange mix

Sprinkle on black pepper

Broil Chops 2 minutes

Turn over

Garnish with more Orange mix

Broil chops for 2 more minutes

Roasted Veggies

Ingredients:

1 lb. Peeled yellow squash – cut in ¾ inch cubes

4 tablespoons soy sauce

2 small chopped onions

6 sliced fresh mushrooms

2 peeled carrots cut into thin 2 inch slices

1 packet Stevia or Splenda

2 teaspoons peanut oil

Dash of Tabasco Sauce

¼ cup sugar free Orange marmalade

2 teaspoons Orange Juice

1 teaspoon Worsteshire sauce

Directions:

Place cubes of squash, mushrooms, carrots and onions in a lightly oiled baking dish.

In a bowl combine Marmalade, Orange juice, soy sauce, peanut oil, sweetener and Worsteshire sauce - liberally garnish the mix over veggies

Bake @ 450 for 20 minutes, stirring occasionally

General Tso's Shrimp and Veggies

Ingredients:

1 pint of General Tso's sauce (from Chinese take out store)

1/8 head of Cabbage cut into one inch chunks

12 uncut medium mushrooms

1 package of Tofu, drained and cut into 1 inch cubes

1/3 medium onion sliced

3 asparagus spears cut into thirds

1 peeled carrot cut into 6 -8 slices

1 small eggplant sliced into ¼ inch pieces

8 frozen jumbo shrimps pre cooked

Directions:

Place everything into a baking dish.

Garnish liberally with General Tso's sauce.

Bake @ 450 for ten minutes

Seriously Chunky Vegetable Creamy Tofu Spread

Ingredients:

8 oz of Tofu Cream Spread (like cream cheese made with Tofu) which is available in most health food stores or in any bagel shop.

1 stalk of celery

1 small onion

½ red bell pepper

1 raw broccoli stem (not the florets; just the stem)

Small amount julliene carrots

Three medium sized walnuts

Directions:

Chop up all of the veggies and walnut with a sharp knife.

Mix with the cream Tofu spread.

Chill for an hour.

Sprinkle minced garlic on a small bagel or a small whole-grain pita and toast.

Serve toasted bagel or pita with Vegetable creamy Tofu spread

Eleven

Okay, you've finished dinner and perhaps now you're craving a bit of dessert or a late night snack? Here are a few suggestions.

Fat-free, sugar-free low-carb Jell-O instant chocolate pudding, 4 – 6 oz, served with a few chopped walnuts or almond slivers and covered with a little whipped cream. This instant pudding mix also comes in butterscotch, white chocolate and vanilla as well.

Low-carb vanilla yogurt, 4 oz, with a few chopped walnuts, either served alone or covered with a thin topping of the instant low-carb chocolate pudding listed above.

Low-carb cheesecake, available in the frozen section of some supermarkets.

Low-carb granola cereal, 4 oz, with a *very* small sprinkling of raisins; covered with skim milk or reduced fat milk. It requires no sweetener, but you can add one packet, or less, if you like.

Another option is two to three low-carb cookies, which are available in health stores. Beware of certain "low-carb" cookies now being sold in the cookie section of your supermarket. Many of them, as of this writing, contain partially hydrogenated oils with trans-fatty acids.

Low-carb pound cake, 4 oz.

Cakes and cookies can be taken with a glass of skim or low fat milk.

Low-carb ice cream, 4 oz.

One low-carb candy bar, usually available in health food stores; Each 4 oz bar can contain up to 220 calories but the carbs are pretty low.

In case you were wondering, you may have only *one single* dessert each day, *or* one late night snack, but not both.

Well, that's about it. I hope that you've enjoyed reading about my personal experiences with dieting, drinking, exercise, supplements and the like. Of utmost importance, I hope that you can derive some real benefits from my own experiences and from "A Diet For The Beer-Drinking Man".

When I write "of utmost importance", *I mean it*. True, I wanted to write this book and hopefully sell a million copies. But for me an equally compelling reason was to be able to bring, what I feel to be, the priceless benefits of my own dieting experiences to the millions of guys out there, who like me, could never manage to successfully lose weight and keep it off.

LISTINGS FOR MEAL SELECTIONS

In reviewing the following listings, please bear in mind the following points:

(1)   The number just to the right following the selection (shown in parenthesis) is the number of choices that this particular food counts for. For breakfast and lunch you should attempt to keep the total number of choices to two; for dinner no more than three.

(2)   When I mention mayonnaise, margarine or cream cheese, I recommend that you use the products that are made using expeller-pressed oils, which contain no trans-fatty acids or partially hydrogenated oils. There are several available these days, in many supermarkets and most easily obtained at health food stores.

(3)   If I list a sandwich as a choice, it assumes that you will use either a low-carb bread or wrap. Light bread is also fairly low in carbs.

(4)   Concerning bread on the side, this assumes two slices of low carb or light bread, or five saltine crackers or three slices of Melba toast.

BREAKFAST CHOICES

Total number of choices should be no more than (2).

Low fat cottage or farmer's cheese, 4 oz. (1)

or

Any cheese, not high in fats, 3 thin slices. (1)

or

Ham or Turkey, 3 thin slices. (1)

or

Low carb yogurt, 4 oz. (1)

or

Low carb (high fiber) bran cereal, 1/3 cup before adding skim milk. (1)

or

Low carb bread or toast with margarine, one slice. (1/2)
[2 slices= choice]

or

Hard boiled egg whites, 6 eggs. (1)

or

Scrambled or fried eggs, egg whites or fat-free egg substitute. (1)

or

Egg, egg-white or fat-free egg substitute omelet mixed with any of the following; mushrooms, onions or acceptable veggies. (1)

or

Same omelet as above but with 2-3 slices of low fat cheese or thin slices of ham or turkey. (2)

or

Tuna, egg or seafood salad with expeller-pressed oil mayonnaise, 4 oz. (1)

and

Coffee or tea with a small amount of milk and sugar-free substitute. (0)

LUNCHEON SELECTIONS

Total number of choices should be no more than (2). Please bear in mind that If I list a sandwich as a choice, it assumes that you will use either a low-carb bread, pita or wrap. Light bread is also fairly low in carbs. You may have any sugar-free drink you desire.

Sandwich with tuna, egg, chicken or seafood salad, with lettuce and one thin slice of tomato. (2)

or

Sandwich with 2-3 slices (any combination, not exceeding 2-3 slices) of ham, turkey, baloney or low fat cheese; with mayo or mustard. (2)

or

Sandwich with salted fried egg whites, or broiled eggplant plus lettuce and mayo. (2)

or

Hamburger or grilled white meat chicken with onion, one thin slice of tomato and low-carb ketchup. (2)

or

Cheeseburger or grilled white meat chicken burger, made as above, one (single) slice of low fat cheese. (2)

or

1 cup of chicken or beef broth, French onion or miso soup, plain or with fresh spinach and 1 oz of soft tofu. You may add a side order of 2 slices of low carb bread. (2)

or

A traditional medium salad, with a plethora of lettuce and low-carb greens. No tomatoes, croutons, or beans. You may chop up 2 slices of low fat cheese, ham or turkey if you wish (any combination, totaling 2 slices) and enjoy 1 slice of low carb bread and a cup of plain broth on the side. Oil and vinegar is the best dressing, but any low carb dressing will do.(2)

or

Pizza; on 1 low carb wrap or 2 halves of pita, spread pizza sauce and sprinkle with mozzarella cheese and bake until cheese is crisp. 2 slices. (2)

DINNER CHOICES

For dinner your total number of choices should be no more than (2 1/2). You can also use any sugar-free drink you desire.

Hamburger, Cheeseburger or Grilled Chicken burger as specified in luncheon selections. (2)

or

Traditional medium salad as specified in luncheon selections. (2)

or

Negemaki, made with scallion pieces, rolled in slices of flank steak and broiled in soy sauce, lemon juice and wine with a few packets of sweetener

or

Tempura shrimp, salmon, beef, chicken, pork or veggies (2)

or

Teriyaki steak, chicken, pork, salmon, tuna or shrimp (2)

or

Filet Mignon with Cognac sauce; cognac, mixed with barbecue sauce (2)

or

Balsamic Steak; Filet Mignon garnished in Balsamic Vinegar, with lemon, Dijon mustard, horseradish and sweetener (2)

or

Honey Mustard Glazed Chicken in a sauce of honey, Dijon mustard, lemon juice and sweetener (2)

or

Whole grain or low carb pasta, 1 oz before boiling. Add lobster, clam, marinara or any Italian sauce. Or simply use oil and vinegar and parmesan cheese. (2)

or

Ziti made with whole grain or low carb ziti or penne noodles, mixed with red Italian sauce, fresh mushrooms and zucchini; topped with low fat shredded mozzarella cheese; Bake until cheese is at desired crispness. (2)

or

Eggplant slices with added sliced mushrooms, zucchini & onions, topped with red Italian sauce and low fat shredded mozzarella cheese; baked. (2)

or

A bowl of chicken or beef broth, french onion or miso soup, plain or with plenty of fresh spinach, sliced mushrooms and 3 oz of soft tofu. You may add a side order of 2 slices of low carb bread. (2)

or

Chicken breast with quasi rice, broth mix and veggies (no corn, tomato, beans or beets). (2)

or

Soft tofu cubes or eggplant slices (4-6 z.) with mushrooms, onions, carrots, & cabbage chunks; broiled with a light garnishing of General Tso's sauce or peanut sauce, brown gravy or barbeque sauce. (1)

or

Pepper steak: Beef chuck, boiled in 1-2 inches of water and beef broth until very tender. Served with brown gravy, cooked onions, mushrooms and blanched green pepper slices, over quasi rice or low carb thin spaghetti noodles. (2)

or

Beef with broccoli: chuck steak prepared as above, except served with cooked broccoli florets, mushrooms, onions and julienne carrots. (2)

or

Barbequed spareribs: spareribs or slices of pork, garnished with sweet & sour sauce or General Tso's or barbeque sauce, broiled until crisp. (2)

or

Egg rolls; Canned bean sprouts, fresh mushrooms, onions, sliced cabbage & scrambled fat free eggs; rolled in low carb wrap and broiled until outside is crispy; or deep-fried until brown. (1)

or

Fried rice; Same ingredients as egg rolls, except with added pre-fried quasi-rice (rice substitute) and no low carb wrap. (1)

or

Lo Mein: Same ingredients as egg rolls, except with low carb spaghetti noodles, no eggs, no wrap, served with brown gravy. (1)

or

Calzone; 1 part shredded mozzarella to 1 part cottage cheese. With added sausage or ham slices, green pepper & onions, rolled & baked in a low carb wrap; or deep fried until brown. (2)

or

Meat or fish, up to 8 oz cooked any fashion. (1)

or

Veggies up to 8 oz. (1)

or

Low carb bread, 2 slices with margarine. (1)

or

Chicken or beef broth with mushrooms and veggies; with tofu or eggplant slices, or with low carb noodles or quasi-rice. (1)

or

Anything from **"Specialty Recipes"** section. (2 1/2)

INDEX TO RECIPES

Afterword

Endnotes by Lisa Cosman, Nutritionist

Now that you've enjoyed reading your way through Roger's Diet Book, I have some observations for you.

Remember, *A Diet For The Beer-Drinking Man IS a Diet;* you need to learn what to do. This worked for Roger because he made some consistent changes in his daily routine that eliminated some old foolish eating habits. Roger told me about his eating habits before his dieting exploration began. After the Marines, he was somewhat casual about exercising and he often didn't eat all day long. Both of those all-too-human Bad Health Habits lead to overeating at night and probably led to Roger's original guzzling (his word) of up to four beers a day...which he got to like so well that he eventually built a whole diet around them. (Someone else might simply have overeaten, or binged on sweets.) Roger liked (he tells us) beer and pasta.

Roger (as you know from his odyssey) had some disturbing experiences with the usual Low Carbohydrate Diet Plans (deprivation followed by binging). He had enough sense to realize that the published Low Carbohydrate Diets weren't going to work for him because his blessed beer was forbidden.

He thought it over, he decided to design a diet for himself.

He factored in the carbohydrates in beer and began to cut them out elsewhere. Once he discovered that the world offered a number of low-carb substitutes, he freed himself to become creative.

Ultimately, what he created was a Controlled Carbohydrate Eating Plan.

It includes beer.

Roger stopped skipping meals.

He prioritized a form of exercise (riding his bicycle) that he likes, and he built up to a consistent exercise schedule.

He began to shop for low-carbohydrate substitutes, and experimented with the recipes he knew until he came up with some very creative substitutes of his own. He discovered that he could finally diet without deprivation!

Why did this diet work for Roger? Why is it likely to work for you if you are a guy who enjoys beer as much as Roger does? (There is too much beer in this diet for women, for a number of reasons; this is specifically a diet for guys.) (More on the amount of alcohol and alternatives, in a bit.)

There is consistent exercise. Don't expect this diet to work unless you begin and build a regular program of exercise you enjoy. It need not be a bicycle; pick what you like, Roger likes the bicycle and dislikes the gym; I, for one, enjoy the gym but one that includes a good lap pool; some people are serious runners or serious walkers, other take dance classes. *The important thing is to discover a safe exercise that you enjoy. And be sure to start slowly and get your doctor's approval, especially if you are currently a couch potato.*

There are three meals a day.

There are lots of low-glycemic, low carbohydrate vegetables (didn't your mother tell you -- or a teacher, or a friend, or a nutritionist or doctor -- to Eat More Vegetables?)

Roger keeps regular hours and gets enough sleep.

There is portion control; he retrained his appetite

There is Structure....and Roger has a Life..

Ultimately, you may (most people do) put into Roger's Diet some creative solutions of your own, to cover your own food favorites. Just remember to keep the carbohydrates under control, but *not too low*; you are going to exercise, and you need to fuel your muscles as well as your heart and your brain.

However, bear in mind that Roger has structured this so that you can simply begin with his plan. It worked for him: his blood pressure, his cholesterol, and his weight all came down (I insisted he show me his medical records).

For the length of a Diet (Six months? Nine months? A year?) this appears to be safe as well as effective. Still, Roger's body (apart from his beer drinking) is not your body. We all can tell if we are overweight. If we are truthful, we also know if we have poor eating habits. Still, get blood work from your doctor, have a discussion, have your cholesterol and your blood pressure checked (besides, you and your doctor will then have something to measure against besides your scale, later)....

Once you have taken off the weight, and regularized your daily food habits, you can address some of the things I dislike about some of Roger's choices.

So what are my reservations?

Roger suggests (sometimes in passing; sometimes consistently) some foods that are disturbingly high in sodium: soy chips (even the low salt ones taste dreadfully salty to me); Chinese Take Out Sauces (MSG and salt); bouillion cubes, powdered beef broth and condensed broths (MSG and salt); (*there are MSG-free and sodium free canned broths available*); powdered steak seasoning, gravies, "liquid smoke" (MSG and salt); you may discover others in your own kitchen (once you get into this diet, become a label reader). Look for low-sodium soy sauce.

Surprisingly enough, even so, Roger's blood pressure came down. I assume it was because he ate lots and lots of fresh vegetables which are high in potassium, he exercised regularly and seriously, and drank lots of water (four to six glasses a day). A good thing, too, since beer (and coffee) is dehydrating.

He also enjoys sour cream and cream cheese. Be sure to purchase low fat sour cream (NOT non-fat sour cream; non-fat sour cream is flavorless). Buy either Neufchatel cheese (which has been around, chemical-free, for decades) as your low-fat cream cheese, or check your local low-fat cream cheese label and be sure it is chemical additive and preservative free (ascorbic acid is fine, that is vitamin C).

Roger is permissive about artificial sweeteners (I'm not). If you've a beer allowance, trust me, you can do without diet sodas. If you want non alcoholic fizz, drink seltzer; if plain seltzer bores you, have a slice of lemon or lime with it. To avoid the artificial sweetener in Roger's Vegetable Juice Cocktail, don't sweeten it. Use the water to extend the tomato vegetable juice and thin it out, and replace the bottled lemon juice with the juice of two or three fresh lemons. Roger's recipe needs sweetening because he uses so very much concentrated lemon juice.

Roger even suggests some fried and deep fried foods. "Fried" is the ultimate "F" word to a nutritionist. Major unhealthy. Anything "fried" can be either baked or grilled. Try it.

He still flours some foods (a step down from breading, granted). Flouring is unnecessary, and although it adds "only a bit of carbohydrate" actually blurs the flavor of foods. Skip it..

There is not a structured amount of oil in this diet. *Just as we need carbohydrates and water, vegetables and proteins, exercise and sufficient sleep, we need healthy fat.* Allow yourself two or three Tablespoonsful of healthy oil every day (you'll burn it off exercising). Remember, although this is a diet for men, not women, both men and women need good fat for our hormone system, our brains, to absorb fat soluble nutrients (including E, A, D, and Calcium). Divide the daily allowance over at least two of your three meals. Chose extra virgin olive oil, expeller pressed high oleic safflower oil, or regular safflower oil mayonnaise (buy oils without preservatives and store them in the refrigerator to prevent even subtle rancidity). (Rancid fats destroy E in the body.)

Remember that there are three teaspoonsful in each Tablespoonful of oil; use on lettuce or in your recipes. Your body will work better, and your skin will be more supple. Olive oil and high oleic safflower oil and safflower mayonnaise help to lower total cholesterol and bad cholesterol but protect good cholesterol.

Roger is a bit egg-yolk phobic. (There was a fanatic fear of egg yolks in the 1970's; new research demonstrates that the real egg/cholesterol problem lies in the bacon/sausage/ham fat on the griddles in which eggs are often cooked.) You can usually find high omega-3 flax-fed eggs in natural food stores (they are fresher and taste better, too), and omega 3's metabolize cholesterol. Indeed, half of the protein in an egg is in the yolk, as well as the Zinc, Zeaxanthin, and Biotin. Just stay away from the ham, the bacon, and the sausage.

Roger is right about the value of low fat cheeses; he also likes some "veggie" cheeses (he says the provolone and the pepper jack). I find "veggie" cheeses unpleasant, but you might like these. However, read the labels very carefully, I could only locate one brand that was all natural; most have a long list of chemical colorings, additives, and preservatives; read the labels carefully.

Once you reach a full exercise level, you could include some low glycemic index, low carbohydrate fruits (just not sweet fruits or fruit juices). Look at grapefruit, strawberries, and kiwi. Fruits (like raw lettuce salads) cleanse the system, add healthy fresh food fiber, and provide additional vitamins and minerals.

Please note that Roger (page 46) points out that he does not smoke. If you do smoke, stop. You know it's bad for you (and dangerous for your heart and, as second hand smoke, for those who love you).

Roger needs a bit of guidance with his multivitamin suggestions. Beta Carotene was originally perceived as a safe form of vitamin A. No more. Recent research (Scandinavian) discovered that it is, actually, potentially dangerous. Carotenoid researchers a few years ago discovered that when the predominate A is Beta Carotene, it blocks the receptor sites in the body for all of the other essential carotenoids (lutein, lycopene, zeaxanthin, et al). So look for a comprehensive multiple with significantly mixed carotenoids and a nice balance of the B's (but no more than 100 mcg. of B12; too much B12 obliterates folic acid AND increases appetite). Your E should have both all of the tocopherols and all of the tocotrienols (you'll need a serious health food store to locate both the comprehensive multiple and a full quality vitamin E). Ester C is fine (I was a fortunate guest at the NYCity presentation of the original research). Ester C is trademarked, and mostly, also a health store available product.

Men get osteoporosis, too. Roger is overcautious about his calcium numbers. Ask your healthfood store for a Calcium/Magnesium formula whose label dosage delivers 500 mg. of Calcium and 250 mg of Magnesium in a day's supply (preferably as a dependable amino acid complex) (this leaves enough room for the cheese calcium and green vegetable magnesium in Roger's diet plan).

Those are my reservations.

My further suggestions? Expand Roger's vegetable suggestions to include zucchini, swiss chard, bok choy and other green leafy vegetables (take a stroll through your local farmer's market in the summer). Remember that cucumbers are an excellent *very* low carbohydrate vegetable, delicious and convenient (peel if waxed, as they usually are in supermarkets). Try adding romaine and other raw lettuces to your menu, use part of your oil allowance to make a simple, Classic Dressing: 1 Tablespoon of oil to 1 teaspoon of wine vinegar or cider vinegar; a ¼ teaspoon of Dijon mustard or one minced clove of garlic, a ¼ teaspoon of dried thyme or oregano or dill leaves, a pinch of salt, a few grinds of black pepper. Fork blend: it's easy, it is delicious.

Explore low-calorie (therefore low-carb) wholegrain crackers, et al.

About those four beers a day... ...

Apparently three or four beers a day are typical for a beer drinking guy. That is the entrance to the rest of this Beer Drinking Diet for guys. Eventually, Roger (and the rest of you guys) really should drop that down to two beers. I'd suggest one of the low carb beers or light beers (Roger flirts with these, then backs off). When dieting, you might as well cut non-essential calories as well as limiting carbohydrates. I'll remind you that current research says that non-alcoholic adult men are safe with 2 beers a day, or two glasses of wine. Beers means 12 ounce bottles, wine means 4-6 ounce glasses. I really doubt the safety of hard liquor (vodka, rum, etc); people behave differently on hard liquor, and often (nowadays) end up drinking strange, oversize cocktails. Stick with the beer or wine, they are closer to food.

This diet is not for alcoholics, children, pregnant or nursing women, children, or the elderly.....all of whose nutrient needs preclude and warn against beer (or other) drinking.

To wind up with some compliments:

Look at the following recipes, they are unique and they will probably amuse you as well as nourish you:

Quasi Mashed Potatoes (use safflower oil; skip the margarine) *(pg. 57), Olive Oil Steaks (pg.63), Baked Eggplant (pg. 64 and pg. 76), Egg Drop Soup (pg. 86), and Stuffed Skirt Steak (pg. 90).*

Remember, Roger's whole idea is to diet without feeling deprived. So, enjoy the process. Let him know about your success.

Sincerely,

Lisa Cosman,

Nutritionist

New York City, 2006